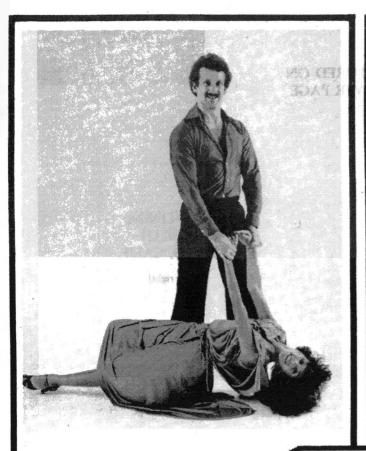

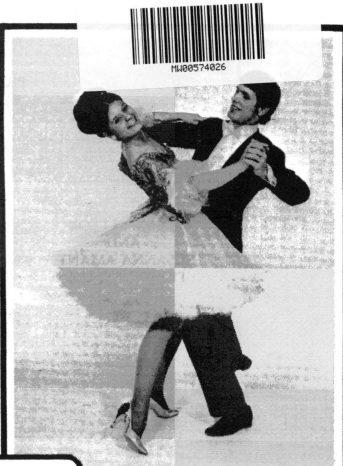

THE DANCERS
(see next page)

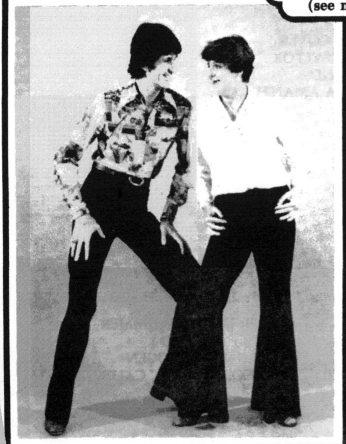

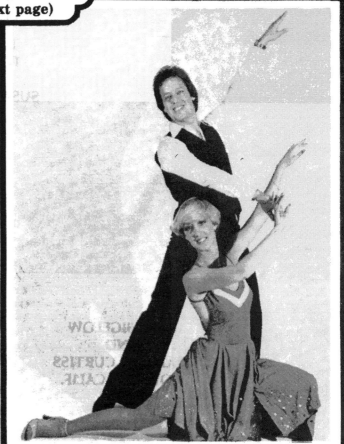

PICTURED ON
COVER PAGE

**TOM MATTOX
AND
SUSANNA AMANTI
DOWNEY, CALIF.**

(upper left)

**LEE AND LINDA
WAKEFIELD
MODESTO, CALIF.**

(upper right)

COLOR
COVER PHOTOS

FRONT COVER
SKIPPY BLAIR

BACK COVER
TOM MATTOX
AND
SUSANNA AMANTI

**CLIFF BIGELOW
AND
MARILYN CURTISS
DOWNEY, CALIF.**

(lower left)

**BUDDY SCHWIMMER
AND
LYNN VOGEN
COSTA MESA, CALIF.**

(lower right)

to John & Jean –
We've come a long way in
from Arthur Murray's at
1955. Dancers are young at
heart – Forever !
God Bless
and have
a great
life !

Skippy

Skippy
Blair

2ND PRINTING
BY POPULAR DEMAND

DISCO TO TANGO
and BACK

PLUS

TEACHER'S BREAKDOWN
for the

UNIVERSAL
UNIT SYSTEM

Copyright Page

DISCO to TANGO and BACK
PLUS
A complete Teacher's Text Covering the
UNIVERSAL UNIT SYSTEM ®
Copyright 1978 -- 2007 by Skippy Blair. All rights reserved.

Library of Congress Catalog #78-73049
ISBN #0-932980-015

Chapter I and II contain the revised entire text of Skippy Blair's "Dance Experience Notebook." "Copyright 1974 by Skippy Blair. Library of Congress Catalog # A-674-188."

"Also included are revised parts of "So You Want to Learn to Dance?" Copyright 1964.

Official Dance Text Book for the 𝕲𝖔𝖑𝖉𝖊𝖓 𝕾𝖙𝖆𝖙𝖊 𝕯𝖆𝖓𝖈𝖊 𝕿𝖊𝖆𝖈𝖍𝖊𝖗𝖘 𝕬𝖘𝖘𝖔𝖈𝖎𝖆𝖙𝖎𝖔𝖓 (GSDTA)
National Headquarters, Downey, CA.

Below is the current contact information for the 2007 printing.
for **Dance Dynamics** ® -
𝕲𝖔𝖑𝖉𝖊𝖓 𝕾𝖙𝖆𝖙𝖊 𝕯𝖆𝖓𝖈𝖊 𝕿𝖊𝖆𝖈𝖍𝖊𝖗𝖘 𝕬𝖘𝖘𝖔𝖈𝖎𝖆𝖙𝖎𝖔𝖓 ® -
and the *World Swing Dance Council*

**Updates on the Universal Unit System are available online at:
www.Swingworld.com
Skippy Blair's entire "Dance Terminology Notebook" (value $40)
is also available on that website Free of charge.
To contact the author personally, email: Skippy@Skippyblair.com**

GSDTA Office Hours: Weekdays 11am to 3pm: 562-869-8949

PREFACE

To the 2nd Printing By *Skippy Blair*

Please Read This First

This 2nd Printing has been by demand of dance organizations and colleges who use this book as their fundamental "Dance Text." Quoting Amazon.com: *"Disco to Tango* has now become a collectors item and is selling for over $100 a copy."

A new GSDTA text, already in the works, will probably not be available for another one or two years. (The original took five.) In the meantime, this 2nd printing, 2007, contains a few corrections and updated entries on:

"Rolling Count" - "Salsa" - "West Coast Swing."

Please see the Copyright Page (page IV) in the front of the book for local contact information.

GSDTA is an Educational Association, known for developing exceptional degrees of coordination, balance and body control, as well as musicality. The result is always a greater degree of understanding and better dance performances. A few dedicated dancers achieve certification status through GSDTA. All are accomplished through the study of

"Dance Dynamics®" and the "Universal Unit System.(R)"

Here's the original Preface from 1978. Still sounds great to me: *Skippy Blair,* **2007:**

This is not your average, *read from start to finish* text book. Use it in different ways:
1. Reading just the Terminology Section takes you on an exciting adventure in dance.
2. Finding specific dances to explore, gets you out on the dance floor.
3. Chapter I and II provide a real "Hands-On" (Feet & Body On) dance experience.
4. Like good food or good music, it takes time to digest the printed material offered in this book. Don't rush through it. Take time to enjoy the process.
5.The theories and drills described in this book can help you reach your highest potential.   In order to do that, you must accept the responsibility of the Study - the Practice = and the actual Mileage that is necessary to produce a really good dancer or a really good teacher. I know that you can do it.

FOREWORD

By Ken Harper

It was not until I met Skippy that I found not only a method, but a person who could give one a theoretical base for all dance: the Universal Unit System. Indeed, different dance teachers are noted for their individual capabilities, but she puts them all together.

Recently, I have opened my own Center, using the Universal Unit System. The rapidity with which the student learns and retains the material makes me envious when I think of all the time and money I invested in learning a few steps by the old "rote" method.

This book is a product of an author who possesses an inner source of energy. To be around her is to capture the energy of the Universe. If you will read and study this book with awareness, you will do more than learn a few dance steps. You will experience her energy. I would have liked to have called the book "The Inner Game of Dance." As with all creative minds and performers, it is their inner energy which makes the difference. In my lifetime, I am sure that I will never know anyone as devotedly dedicated and totally unselfish and "giving" of her inner self.

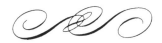

• Dr. Kenneth Harper has acquired four degrees: B.A./M.A./B.D./ & a PH.D. in Psychology, Sociology, Anthropology and Philosophy.

His career in public education has been one of service:
   . . . as SUPERINTENDENT OF SCHOOLS in South Rhodesia, Africa . . .
   . . . as DEAN of the University of Kentucky . . .
   . . . as PRESIDENT of TWO COLLEGES . . . Pima and Riverside . . .

His love of the dance has led him to study for and achieve teacher status in the field of Social Dance as well as Dance Therapy. His desire to "work with the people" led him to opening his own "CENTER" in Riverside. Ken is also a member of G.S.D.T.A.

FOREWORD

By John Buckner

To analyze the authority of the author, we would have to trace her dance history back to specific eras.

When "Swing" was the competition dance most widely known, Skippy was developing Swing dancers at both amateur and professional level that took home the prizes. When Latin competitions developed, she again produced top quality dancers & winners.

While other teachers waited for the Twist to die a natural death, Miss Blair developed a curriculum that teachers nationwide used as a standard. With the emergence of Rock and Solo dancing, once more her dancers stood out in shows, competitions and as teachers. Her Rock curriculum was developed starting in 1968 and gained momentum in 1971. By 1973 it had become a standard and those basics are still in evidence today, as teachers adopt their own version of the original. By 1975 and '76 "touch" dancing and Disco were on the scene, as predicted by Skippy in 1971.

One of her talents lies in being able to recognize a "trend" and being able to identify what she calls the "essence" of each new dance. With this analysis comes her ability not only to teach and to train other teachers but also to record for posterity those forms of dance that will endure.

To my knowledge Skippy is one of the top contemporary dance analysts in the country today. It doesn't take much discussion to realize that this superior "Lady of the Dance" knows of which she speaks. Her graphic descriptions of competition dancers or performers and their best points and their worst points makes the dancer emerge in a new light. Her identification of the problem areas are not only educational to the listener, but serve as a wealth of learning for those who ask for constructive criticism.

I feel honored to have been involved in the development of this new and exciting breakthrough in dance education. The contents of this book will truly revolutionize the entire teaching field in all areas of dance.

- John Buckner started his dancing career with Calls Fine Arts in Long Beach some 25 years ago. He spent several years at the Skippy Blair Studios in Downey, during which time he appeared in numerous shows and spent a great deal of time winning dance contests. Later John fulfilled a lifelong dream by working for DISNEYLAND. Recently, he returned to his first love . . . the DANCE and re-joined the family of G.S.D.T.A.

John teaches evening dance classes in the Anaheim area and children's classes in the school in the daytime. No doubt his sincere interest in the people he teaches contributes to his success.

INTRODUCTION TO LEARNING . . .

How many times have you watched someone dance and wanted to be able to CATCH whatever they were doing? With the knowledge of the UNITS you would READ what they were doing . . . and more times than not, you would find that what you SAW was merely a RHYTHM VARIATION or a STYLE VARIATION of something you already know.

There is NOTHING quite as exciting as being able to LISTEN to MUSIC and then CONFIDENTLY express your FEELINGS to that Music through DANCE.

Good Dancers are POPULAR PEOPLE. They get more fun out of Life! The poise and confidence that belongs to a good dancer goes far beyond the dance floor.

This book was written for every single person who has ever wanted to learn to dance . . . or ever wanted to IMPROVE the dancing they already do.

To THE BEGINNER DANCER . . . You will gain a BASIC UNDERSTANDING of GOOD DANCING and what it can do for you. Don't be impatient with yourself and don't expect to understand ALL that you read on the first try. Each person should read and study ONLY to the point where they cease to understand. Then . . . START OVER AGAIN from the beginning.

To the ACTIVE STUDENT OF DANCE . . . The material in this book will add to the things you have already learned and help you to understand MANY things that you will learn in the future. Return to the contents AGAIN and AGAIN and you will find something NEW . . . EVERY TIME!

To the TEACHER OF DANCE . . . Along with the countless things you already know, the fundamentals of the UNIVERSAL UNIT SYSTEM will EXPAND your teaching enjoyment, increase your knowledge of all dance . . . and MOST important, it will help you discover how VERY MUCH YOU ALREADY KNOW. (More than you realize!)

To the ACCOMPLISHED DANCER, PERFORMER, CONTESTANT . . . Having studied and delved into Dance Theory for many years, it is like "FINDING A PIECE OF GOLD" when I run across some obscure fact, (often right under my nose) that was not obvious to me before. The discovery . . . by YOU . . . of even ONE little "piece of Gold" will make reading this book worthwhile. It is only when we decide that we have nothing left to learn . . . that we cease to grow. But YOU must be the growing type . . . or you wouldn't be READING this book!

To the NON-DANCER . . . YES! . . . YOU TOO will learn a lot of valuable information. ANYTHING that you learn will be more than you knew before. Like GOOD MUSIC . . . It is possible to APPRECIATE good dancing without actually PARTICIPATING. More and more people are being EDUCATED to GOOD DANCING. Today is an ERA of EDUCATION in all fields . . . and SOCIAL DANCE is no exception!

ONE SEMESTER with the UNIVERSAL UNIT SYSTEM equips the student of Dance with the FUNDAMENTALS for ALL FORMS OF DANCE.

If you are a "PATTERN SNATCHER," chances are that you will flip to specific dances and try to interpret the material . . . without ever having gone through the BASIC UNIT STRUCTURE of the system. (See Chapter I & II.) If you do NOT read Chapter I, you are cheating yourself. By studying Chapter I, YOU become the Master of your dancing future. The FUNDAMENTALS that tie ALL DANCE together, are learned in a way that ELIMINATES FAILURE!!

Learning a specific Dance, teaches you only that specific Dance. Learning the COM-PONENTS that make up a specific Dance, teaches you how to RECOGNIZE and therefore DUPLICATE, the Dance forms that you will encounter in the FUTURE!! A student of the UNI-VERSAL UNIT SYSTEM is never "Pigeon-holed into an "Era" of Social Dance, but is capable of keeping UP-TO-DATE in ANY ERA. There is no Generation Gap in the World of Dance, when one is knowledgable in the COMPOSITION of every Dance Form.

Are You a SLOW LEARNER? First, let's ask ourselves, "What IS a Slow Learner?" Many would answer that a SLOW LEARNER is one who does not comprehend readily, the material being taught.

My definition of a SLOW LEARNER is one who has not yet found the method that fits his particular learning pattern.

The UNIVERSAL UNIT SYSTEM takes the learning of Dance OUT of the "Talent only" category and gives EVERYONE the tools which help him become knowledgable in the Art of Dance . . . regardless of any inborn talent.

Through the years, it has been my special privilege to witness time and time again, in-dividuals who were considered to have ZERO TALENT, become the best dancers in their category. Several have become recognized TEACHERS . . . Some have become PERFORMERS (not only locally, but in Las Vegas, New York, etc.) The KEY that unlocks ignorance is KNOWLEDGE. For far too long, dancing has been viewed as something that someone needed a special talent for, in or-der to be able to participate. ALL OF US HAVE SPECIAL TALENTS. We develop those talents in different ways. Some MIMIC OTHERS and thereby achieve some sort of form by being able to duplicate what they see. (This accounts for only 1% of the population.) MOST of us need to UN-DERSTAND what is expected before we can perform the expected. That is where the UNIVER-SAL UNIT SYSTEM comes in. It reduces all of these seemingly complicated dances into a few SIMPLE BASIC RHYTHM PATTERNS and a few BASIC MOVEMENT UNITS. Armed with this knowledge, the student is no longer in awe of the mystery of learning to dance . . . because the MYSTERY HAS BEEN TAKEN OUT.

No one marvels that we can sit down and read a new book as soon as it hits the stands. No one rushes back to school to learn how to read this new book. WHY? . . . Because the book is merely an arrangement and rearrangement of WORDS. Knowing those words has taken the mystery out of reading a book. There is no FEAR of reading a new book . . . because the WORDS are the same old familiar words that make up ALL READING. When a NEW DANCE hits the social horizon, there can be NO FEAR when you know the BASIC UNITS that ALL DANCES contain. There is nothing new under the sun . . . only arrangement . . . and rearrangement. You are about to embark on a learning experience that will be beneficial to you for the rest of your life . . . HAPPY LEARNING!

CONTENTS

Chapters I and II contain the
entire revised text from
The "DANCE EXPERIENCE
NOTEBOOK"

KEY to the
"UNIVERSAL UNIT SYSTEM"

A METHOD OF LEARNING
ALL DANCE

Official Handbook of the "GOLDEN STATE DANCE TEACHERS ASSOCIATION"

Chapter I
LEARNING THE BASICS

CONGRATULATIONS . . . You are about to embark on an exciting adventure into the realm of Dance. No matter what your dancing background, (from zero to professional) . . . you are about to discover the "KEY" that takes the mystery out of learning ALL FORMS OF DANCE . . . EASILY and QUICKLY!!

This important KEY is found in this FIRST CHAPTER and is based on one INCREDIBLE FACT . . . that EVERY PATTERN in EVERY DANCE is composed of arrangements and re-arrangements of THREE PRIMARY RHYTHM UNITS.

FIRST . . . WHAT is a UNIT?

1. A UNIT is | **TWO BEATS OF MUSIC.** |

2. For IDENTIFICATION, | **a UNIT** | is encased in a rectangle.

3. EVERYTHING in that rectangle will refer to those same

| **TWO BEATS OF MUSIC.** |

4. In the BASIC STAGE there are only FOUR PRIMARY UNITS.

5. These PRIMARY UNITS refer to the THREE BASIC RHYTHMS plus a

| **BLANK UNIT.** |

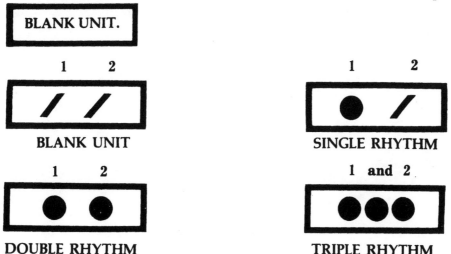

| 1   2 |
| BLANK UNIT |

| 1   2 |
| SINGLE RHYTHM |

| 1   2 |
| DOUBLE RHYTHM |

| 1 and 2 |
| TRIPLE RHYTHM |

1

PRIMARY UNITS

LOOK AT THE UNITS . . . READ from LEFT TO RIGHT what is written UNDER the UNITS.
THEN GET UP AND PRACTICE DANCING from the First Line to the Last.

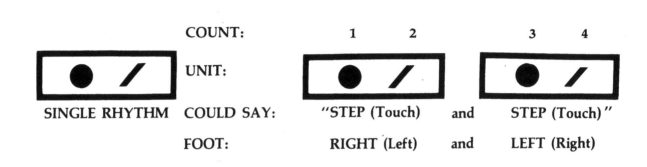

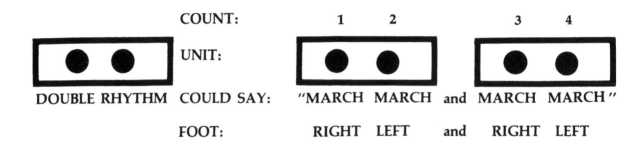

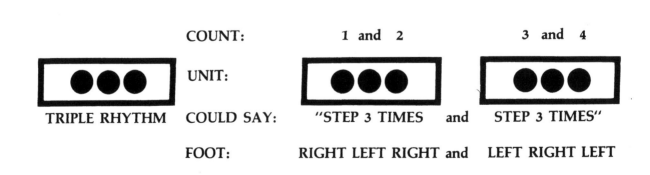

	COUNT:	1	2	3	4
	UNIT:				
BLANK UNIT	COULD SAY:	"(Point Fwd.)	(Point Side)	(Point Back)	(Point Fwd.)"
	FOOT:	(RIGHT)	(RIGHT)	(RIGHT)	(RIGHT)

BLANK

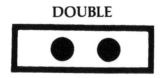

•A BLANK UNIT allows NO weight changes. The same foot will be free at the completion of the unit.

SINGLE   **TRIPLE**

•SINGLE RHYTHM and TRIPLE RHYTHM are interchangeable. Both SINGLE and TRIPLE RHYTHM BEGIN and END on the SAME FOOT. Therefore, we have a "LEFT SINGLE" and a "RIGHT SINGLE" . . . or a "LEFT TRIPLE" and a "RIGHT TRIPLE."

DOUBLE

*•DOUBLE RHYTHM starts on ONE FOOT and ends on the OTHER FOOT . . . either stepping RIGHT/LEFT or stepping LEFT/RIGHT.

---

*For those who have been taught that a "TAP STEP" is DOUBLE RHYTHM: In this new UNIVERSAL UNIT SYSTEM, the "TAP STEP" has not been removed. It has just been recognized as a SECONDARY UNIT, rather than a PRIMARY UNIT. It is now called a DELAYED SINGLE. (see HISTORY AND DEVELOPMENT OF THE UNIVERSAL UNIT SYSTEM).

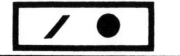

STEP ONCE   ...   STEP TWICE ... OR STEP THREE TIMES ...

SOUND TOO EASY TO BE TRUE ? ...

If you are telling yourself, "I've been doing something like this all along" . . . You are ABSOLUTELY RIGHT!

TEACHERS and STUDENTS of Dance have been doing "SOMETHING LIKE THIS" all along . . . but NOT QUITE!!!

The DIFFERENCE. . . That one thing we have NOT done all along, is have any concrete SYSTEM of passing on the things that take years to learn by experience. The UNIVERSAL UNIT SYSTEM lets you discover the FUNDAMENTALS that OVERLAP into EVERY KNOWN DANCE FORM.

Let's pretend we're back in GRADE SCHOOL and we are about to learn to READ. We know that once we learn to read . . . ALL BOOKS WILL BE OPEN TO US . . . all KNOWLEDGE will be at our fingertips. Well here we are about to learn to "READ" the DANCE . . . and very soon ALL PATTERNS in ALL DANCES will be available to us. READY? Let's go:

To simplify the "reading" we use one large dot [●] to represent a change of weight. Our "reading system" is made up of DOTS and SLASHES. A DOT is a STEP. The SLASH (**/**) means that we do something else on that beat of music. Thus . . . if we STEP on the First beat of the UNIT . . . and so SOMETHING ELSE on the second beat (a [tap] . . . [kick] . . . [touch] . . . etc. with the FREE FOOT) it will be a:

> **SINGLE RHYTHM UNIT.**

What we SAY as we do the STEP PATTERN becomes the VERBAL PATTERN.

A VERBAL PATTERN for | SINGLE RHYTHM | could be | "STEP (touch)" |

| LEFT SINGLE | = STEP on the LEFT FOOT on count ONE and touch the Right foot TO the LEFT FOOT on count TWO.

| RIGHT SINGLE | = STEP on the RIGHT FOOT on count ONE and touch the Left foot to the RIGHT FOOT on count TWO.

| STEP (touch) | = [● **/**] = | SINGLE RHYTHM |

ONE STEP to TWO BEATS OF MUSIC

If we alternate one | LEFT SINGLE | and one | RIGHT SINGLE | we have a
TWO UNIT PATTERN.   Let's DO a TWO UNIT PATTERN.

Select a piece of music that has a medium tempo heavy beat. LISTEN TO THE MUSIC. Count the
beats out loud. You will find that there are FOUR BEATS OF MUSIC to each measure . . . That is
TWO UNITS of the dance. By alternating a LEFT UNIT and a RIGHT UNIT we make a TWO
UNIT PATTERN. Thus we would be dancing to one MEASURE of music .

COUNT: 1   2   3   4   COUNT: 1   2   3   4

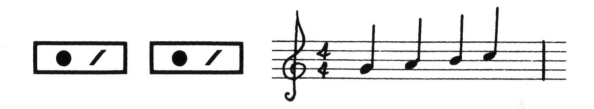

Count out the BEATS of music. Count "One Two Three Four." Now synchronize
that with the VERBAL "Step (touch) Step (touch)" and we will be alternating a

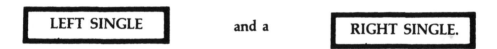

The only thing we have left to complete our STEP PATTERN is DIRECTION. The
use of FOOT POSITIONS eliminates awkward movement before it begins. They
aid in the development of style, balance, form and control. Don't just READ about
them. Look down there at your feet and SEE what they look like on YOU!

1st FOOT POSITION: Feet Together . . . Heels touching. Toes slightly apart.

2nd FOOT POSITION: Feet Directly Apart (Side Step).

3rd FOOT POSITION: Heel to Instep

4th FOOT POSITION: Walking Step . . . Forward or Back

5th FOOT POSITION: Toe to Heel (Back Heel released from the floor.)

SO FAR ... We've done a LEFT SINGLE ... a RIGHT SINGLE ... and we've learned FOUR FOOT POSITIONS ... SHALL WE PUT THOSE TWO TOGETHER? ...

SINGLE RHYTHM   ● /

Let's return now to | SINGLE RHYTHM. | Just by changing the FOOT POSITIONS we can do a variety of patterns. Continue to say:

"STEP (TOUCH)"   "STEP (TOUCH)"   alternating Left and Right SINGLE RHYTHM UNITS ... but vary the foot positions. For example:

STEP in 2nd foot position ... and (TOUCH) in 1st foot position

STEP in 4th ... and (TOUCH) in 3rd

STEP in 1st ... and (TOUCH) in 2nd   The VERBAL PATTERN for

this last one might be   "TOGETHER ... (POINT to the SIDE)"
                                                  1   2

Don't be in too much of a hurry to progress to the next step. Make sure that you can do

SINGLE RHYTHM   in every conceivable way. Do a ("KICK") instead of a (touch)

... making the VERBAL PATTERN: STEP (KICK)   STEP (KICK).

It is still   SINGLE RHYTHM   ...ONE STEP/in a two-beat/ UNIT. It is also possible to

STEP AND (HOLD)   for the second beat (used in all of the LATIN DANCES).

It is still   SINGLE RHYTHM.

LET'S REVIEW. If all of the answers come quickly, we're ready to proceed to the next step. CHECK THESE OUT FIRST:
1. How many beats in a UNIT? _____
2. How many changes of weight in a SINGLE RHYTHM UNIT? _____
3. At the end of a RIGHT SINGLE which foot is free? _____
4. How many UNITS in a measure of 4/4 time? _____

6

DOUBLE RHYTHM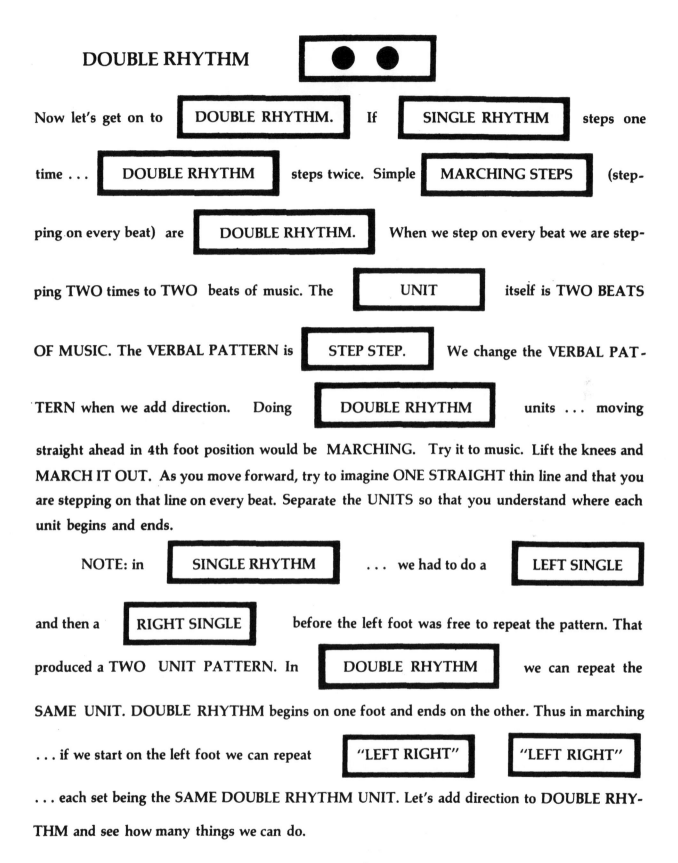

Now let's get on to DOUBLE RHYTHM. If SINGLE RHYTHM steps one time . . . DOUBLE RHYTHM steps twice. Simple MARCHING STEPS (stepping on every beat) are DOUBLE RHYTHM. When we step on every beat we are stepping TWO times to TWO beats of music. The UNIT itself is TWO BEATS OF MUSIC. The VERBAL PATTERN is STEP STEP. We change the VERBAL PATTERN when we add direction. Doing DOUBLE RHYTHM units . . . moving straight ahead in 4th foot position would be MARCHING. Try it to music. Lift the knees and MARCH IT OUT. As you move forward, try to imagine ONE STRAIGHT thin line and that you are stepping on that line on every beat. Separate the UNITS so that you understand where each unit begins and ends.

NOTE: in SINGLE RHYTHM . . . we had to do a LEFT SINGLE and then a RIGHT SINGLE before the left foot was free to repeat the pattern. That produced a TWO UNIT PATTERN. In DOUBLE RHYTHM we can repeat the SAME UNIT. DOUBLE RHYTHM begins on one foot and ends on the other. Thus in marching . . . if we start on the left foot we can repeat "LEFT RIGHT" "LEFT RIGHT" . . . each set being the SAME DOUBLE RHYTHM UNIT. Let's add direction to DOUBLE RHYTHM and see how many things we can do.

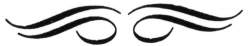

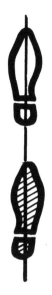

•Thinking FOURTH FOOT POSITION: Step FORWARD on the LEFT FOOT and BACK (in place) on the RIGHT FOOT. This becomes a FORWARD ROCK as done in CHA CHA, TANGO, FOXTROT, RUMBA or SALSA SUAVE.

•Now do the same thing starting with the RIGHT FOOT stepping BACK and the LEFT FOOT FORWARD (in place) producing a BACK ROCK.

•Step SIDE LEFT and bring the feet "together" stepping on the RIGHT FOOT. (2nd foot position to 1st foot position). This produces a "CHASSE'" or "SIDE TOGETHER." Practice moving around the room saying "side together" "side together." Then start with the right foot and travel right.

① ②

Here we go with the questions again.

1. What is a Chasse'? _____

2. A "Side together" consists of which two foot positions?
   _____ & _____

3. If I start with my left foot and complete 3 Double Rhythm Units . . . which foot will be free? _____

4. Can a DOUBLE RHYTHM UNIT replace a SINGLE RHYTHM UNIT? _____

If the answers are easy . . . we are ready to combine these first two units into a step pattern. Don't settle for just any answer. Check your answers out. You are more than half way through your basic "reading" session. So far, the term "RHYTHM" has been used to denote a particular UNIT. (Single, Double, Triple). However, "RHYTHM" is also used to denote a particular RHYTHM PATTERN. For instance: A SINGLE RHYTHM UNIT can be done in many different directions but the underlying recurrent RHYTHM is the same. (STEP on count ONE and do something else on count TWO) . . . and so it is with a RHYTHM PATTERN: A STEP PATTERN (emphasis on the word "STEP") is a series of UNITS that together make up a recognizable "PATTERN." A RHYTHM PATTERN is the foundation for an infinite variety of STEP PATTERNS.

- BOX RHYTHM is a FOUR UNIT PATTERN (8 beats of music)
- BOX RHYTHM alternates SINGLE and DOUBLE RHYTHM UNITS.
- A Step Pattern includes direction and foot positions.

EXAMPLE:

COUNT:	1 2	3 4	5 6	7 8
UNIT:	● ●	● /	● ●	● /
RHYTHM PATTERN:	Double	Single	Double	Single
STEP PATTERN: (in this instance a Box Step)	SIDE TOG.	FWD. (tch)	SIDE TOG.	BACK (tch)
FOOT POSITIONS:	2nd 1st	4th (1st)	2nd 1st	4th (1st)

At this point one is ready to say, "Why didn't you just give the VERBAL PATTERN . . . "Side together Forward and Side together Back . . ."? Simple enough. The VERBAL PATTERN might teach you THIS pattern, but it would not teach you the KEY to more advanced material . . . It would not teach you the UNITS that comprise ALL DANCE.

We are now going to use BOX RHYTHM in several dances. It need not be a BOX STEP. We can do "SIDE TOGETHER" "SIDE (TOUCH)" or we can do "FORWARD TOGETHER" "FORWARD (TOUCH)." Try different combinations in different directions to different types of music.

LATIN DANCES "HOLD" or "DELAY" the second count of the SINGLE RHYTHM UNIT. That means that the "follow thru" or "Touch" happens AFTER count two.

FOXTROT SINGLE RHYTHM UNIT

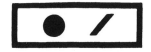

Do a small BOX STEP to the VERBAL PATTERN:

RUMBA SINGLE RHYTHM UNIT

(use RUMBA or DISCO Music)

COUNT:	1	2	3	4*	5	6	7	8*
VERBAL:	Side	Together	Forward	(Hold)	Side	Together	Back	(Hold)
FOOT:	L	R	L		R	L	R	

*(Follow through is on the "&" count after the hold). Add authentic Latin styling by "peeling" the weighted foot from the floor. LIFT the foot from the heel toward the toe. PLACE the foot from the toe to the heel. A SMALL box at first, using correct foot placement and "peel" will produce an automatic Cuban motion. As you do the pattern, look over your left shoulder and you will start turning gradually to the left. Always look in the direction of a turn. Now put on some smooth FOXTROT MUSIC and go back to "touching" or "brushing" one foot past the other on the second count of the unit. Make the FOXTROT smooth and flowing . . . and COUNT OUT the actual beats of the music. THEY MUST MATCH. Our "UNITS" fit into the music like a drum beat. We can't have anything left over. We HAVE to come out EVEN!

If you actually take the time to DANCE all of these things to music, you will be rewarded by your complete understanding of the dance. We are going to do that BOX STEP again . . . but THIS TIME . . . to DISCO MUSIC.

- We have "held" the "follow thru" for RUMBA   (4& . . . 8&)
- We have brushed lightly for FOXTROT   (ON counts 4 . . . 8)
  - Now with DISCO we are going to ACCENT the "follow thru" with a light stamp of the foot on counts 4 and 8.

. . . SAME UNIT STRUCTURE . . . SAME PATTERN . . . DIFFERENT STYLING

At this writing (June 1978) BOX RHYTHM is being danced in CONTEMPORARY FOXTROT and in the TANGO HUSTLE . . . It's the same old BOX STEP, but with a brand new look. Put on some DISCO MUSIC and ACCENT every beat.

COUNT:	1 2	3 4	5 6	7 8
UNIT:	[● ●]	[● /]	[● ●]	[● /]
VERBAL:	"STEP TOGETHER	STEP (stamp)	STEP TOGETHER	STEP (stamp)"
SIDE BASIC:	SIDE TOGETHER	SIDE (stamp)	SIDE TOGETHER	SIDE (stamp)
BOX STEP:	SIDE TOGETHER	FORWARD (stamp)	SIDE TOGETHER	BACK (stamp)

Note that the two patterns above are the SAME RHYTHM PATTERN but are two separate STEP PATTERNS. It is easier to do the SIDE BASIC before doing the BOX STEP. (This is particularly true if you are TEACHING these patterns to groups).

Still staying with the BOX STEP, let's go one step farther. Find a VERY FAST SWING (Charleston tempo) and do a very tiny BOXSTEP using a lilting BOUNCE movement and you will be doing a basic BALBOA. The "touch" in the SINGLE RHYTHM UNIT will be done in 3rd foot position . . . and later you can do a little "kick" in place of the "touch." I hope you are not just READING all of this . . . because it will not mean the same thing as if you are DOING IT.

Time for checking up on what we are learning. If the answers do not come quickly . . . back to the drawing board!

1. How many UNITS IN BOX RHYTHM ? _____

2. How does a RHYTHM PATTERN differ from a STEP PATTERN?
_____

3. In SINGLE RHYTHM we STEP on the first beat of the UNIT. On the SECOND beat which foot position are we in ?
   In RUMBA _____
   In FOXTROT _____
   In BALBOA _____

4. A BOX STEP can start with either a SINGLE or a DOUBLE. No matter WHERE it starts, BOX RHYTHM alternates _____ and _____ RHYTH'

TRIPLE RHYTHM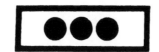

There is only ONE MORE UNIT TO LEARN ... and YOU will be the MASTER of YOUR DANCING FUTURE. "TRIPLE RHYTHM" is just what it sounds like. It "STEPS THREE TIMES" in one UNIT ... that is: THREE STEPS to only TWO BEATS of MUSIC.

If you count the actual beats of the music, you will count:

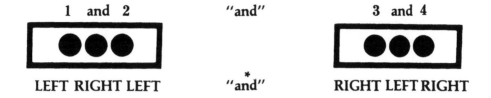

1 and 2	"and"	3 and 4
LEFT RIGHT LEFT	*"and"	RIGHT LEFT RIGHT

That is a repeatable TWO UNIT PATTERN.

SLOW CONTEMPORARY MUSIC is good for practicing TRIPLES. Try them in all different directions. The VERBAL PATTERN could be any of the following: (alternating Left and Right TRIPLES).

LEFT TRIPLE		RIGHT TRIPLE
1 and 2	"and"	3 and 4

VERBAL: "Side Together Side   Side Together Side"

FOOT
POSITION: 2nd 1st 2nd   2nd 1st 2nd

VERBAL: "Side Back Fwd.   Side Back Fwd."

FOOT
POSITION: 2nd 4th 4th   2nd 4th 4th

VERBAL: "Back Fwd. Side   Back Fwd. Side"

FOOT
POSITION: 4th 4th 2nd   4th 4th 2nd

*Lift the Right foot on the "and" between the Units.

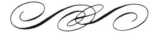

ODD AND EVEN UNITS

No matter how many different ways you vary the direction and/or the foot positions, one thing becomes clear. There are really only TWO KINDS OF UNITS:

•"ODD UNITS" (an odd number of steps: 1, 3, 5, 7 etc.).

TRIPLE RHYTHM and SINGLE RHYTHM require both a LEFT and a RIGHT UNIT to complete a pattern. We can do a LEFT UNIT (begins and ends on left foot) or we can do a RIGHT UNIT (begins and ends on the right foot). One follows the other. These are both ODD UNITS (an odd number of steps).

•"EVEN UNITS" (an even number of steps: 2, 4, 6, 8 etc.).

DOUBLE RHYTHM is complete in itself. You can repeat the same unit over and over again. The same foot is always free. DOUBLE RHYTHM and a BLANK UNIT are the EVEN UNITS.

This "boils down" the UNIT SYSTEM to TWO MAIN UNITS . . . Ones that start with one foot free and end with the OTHER foot free (ODD) . . . and ones that start with one foot free and end with the SAME foot free (EVEN). It is really that simple. THINK ABOUT IT FOR A MOMENT . . . No matter HOW complicated the pattern in ANY DANCE . . . double syncopations . . . hops . . . skips . . . jumps . . . no matter WHAT . . . EVERY PATTERN IN EVERY DANCE can be broken down into these two main kinds of UNITS.

ODD UNITS and EVEN UNITS.

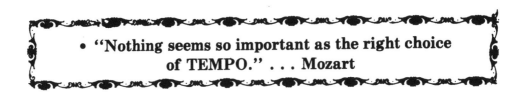

• "Nothing seems so important as the right choice of TEMPO." . . . Mozart

BASIC
FOOT POSITIONS

FIRST FOOT POSITION:

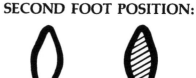

FEET TOGETHER . . . Heels touching
and Toes just SLIGHTLY apart
(about the width of a thumb).

SECOND FOOT POSITION:

FEET DIRECTLY APART . . . A SIDE
Step either to the Left or to
the Right.

THIRD FOOT POSITION: HEEL to INSTEP . . . Back Foot is on an Angle that will allow BOTH knees to face forward when the knees are bent.

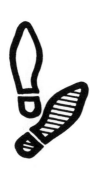

CLOSED THIRD

OPEN THIRD

FOURTH FOOT POSITION: A WALKING STEP . . . Walk a STRAIGHT LINE, with the center of the HEEL and the center of the BIG TOE on the line. Practice with a RIGID Line at first . . . and then picture the LINE as a piece of STRING. It can CURVE in ANY DIRECTION. The CURVE will be in the Direction of the FORWARD FOOT. FORWARD in COUPLES DANCING will be directly under the C.P.B. of ones partner.

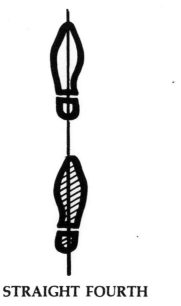

STRAIGHT FOURTH

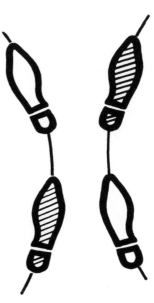

CURVING FOURTH

(See complete chart — end of Chapter II.)

13

GOLDEN WEST BALLROOM
NORWALK, CALIFORNIA
"Dancers have more fun than People!"

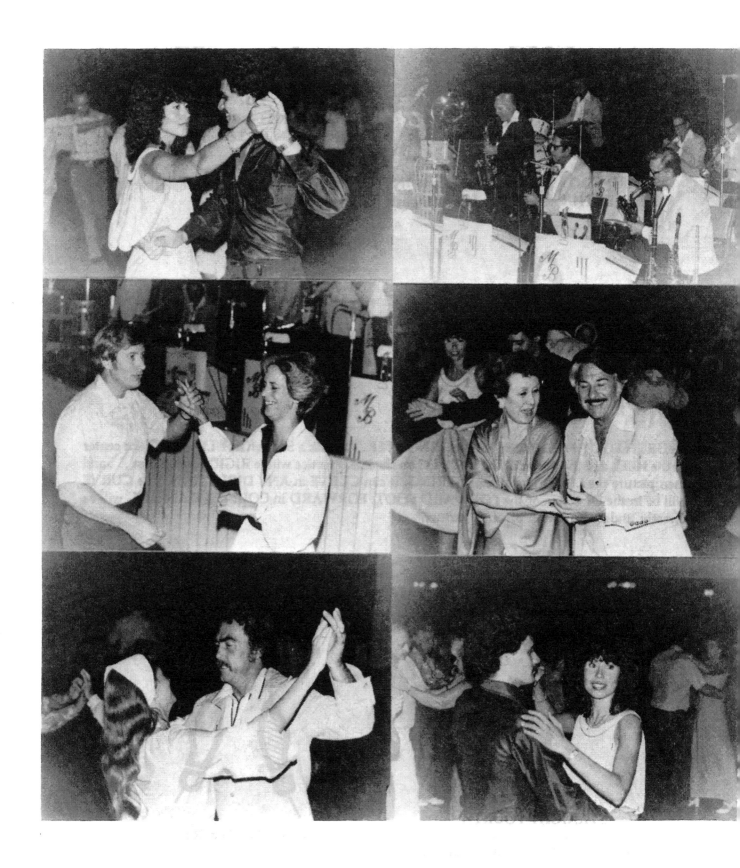

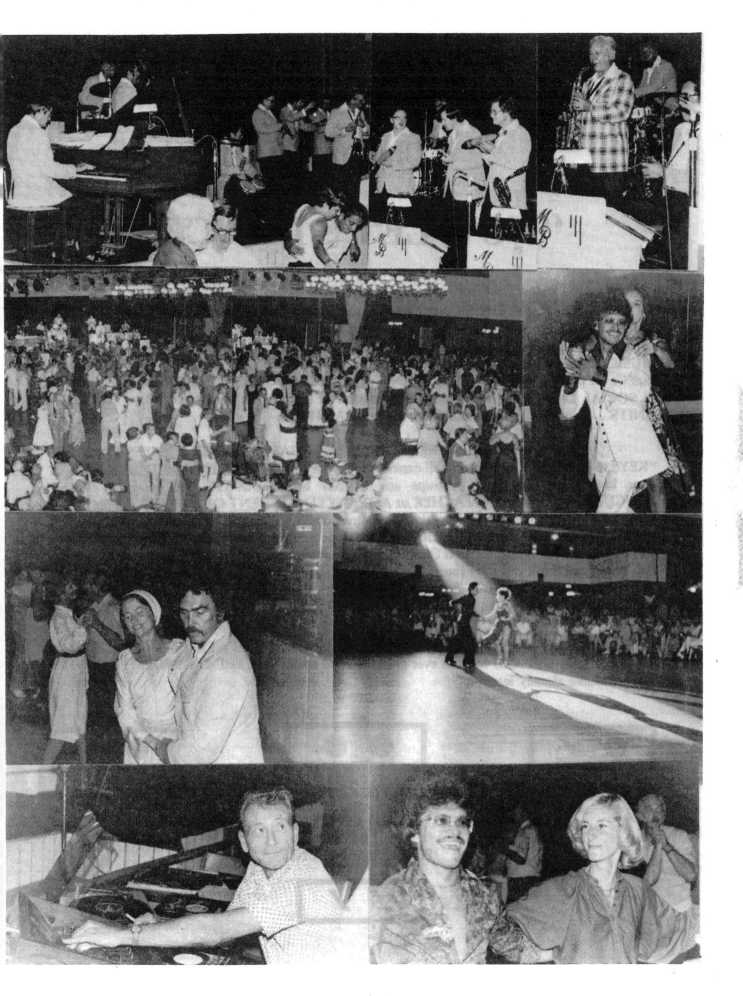

Chapter II

"NOW LET'S DANCE"

The BASIC UNITS that we are dealing with so far are the foundation for ALL PATTERNS IN ALL DANCES. It can be likened to learning MUSIC. We start with four simple quarter notes to a measure . . . and progress from there . . . but no matter HOW COMPLICATED THE MUSIC, the notes will always fit into the measure. The UNIT SYSTEM IS THE SAME . . . except that we are dealing with a TWO BEAT UNIT instead of a FOUR BEAT MEASURE. All Measures of SOCIAL DANCE MUSIC (with the exception of Waltz) can be divided into TWO BEAT UNITS . . . and the UNITS combined, make a PATTERN.

If you have read Chapter I . . . YOU NOW HAVE IN YOUR POSSESSION . . . the "KEY" to learning all variations in all dances. If you are a NEW STUDENT OF THE DANCE . . . your knowledge will grow in leaps and bounds because UNITS will be your "FIRST LANGUAGE." If you are a TEACHER or ADVANCED STUDENT OF DANCE . . . take one of your most intricate patterns and break it down into UNITS. You will be amazed at what you will learn from separating the UNIT PARTS of any given pattern. Remember . . . there IS NO PATTERN that cannot fit into the UNIT SYSTEM . . . just as there is NO MUSIC that cannot be written. When you think you have found the exception . . . accept the fact that there ARE NO EXCEPTIONS and then proceed to figure out HOW it fits. Very soon you will be "READING" the dance steps that you see performed, and creating some of your own.

In SOCIAL DANCE one can perform HUNDREDS of PATTERN VARIATIONS in a VARIETY OF DANCES without ever going beyond the THREE PRIMARY RHYTHM UNITS that you have already learned.

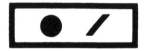   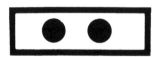   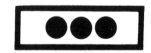

SINGLE RHYTHM . . .   DOUBLE RHYTHM . . .   TRIPLE RHYTHM . . .

PLUS A BLANK UNIT

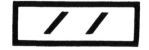

In order to become completely familiar with HOW THE UNITS WORK . . . let's choreograph a simple EIGHT UNIT ROUTINE. That will give us a chance to use ALL of the units we have learned. By making the routine EIGHT UNITS we get a "BONUS." In addition to reenforcing the UNITS we are also learning automatic phrasing. . . . That is . . . if we start with the music . . . right after the introduction . . . we can keep repeating those eight units and we will not only be IN TIME WITH THE MUSIC . . . but will also be ON PHRASE. . . . LISTEN TO THE MUSIC and count the RHYTHM PATTERN AS YOU STEP OUT THE WEIGHT CHANGES IN PLACE. You will begin to FEEL the PHRASE. There is a pause at the end of a phrase just like seeing a period at the end of a sentence. Many intermediate dancers and even some ADVANCED DANCERS have difficulty keeping time to music. STEPPING OUT THE RHYTHM PATTERN before doing the actual STEP PATTERN will eliminate the problem . . . IT WORKS!

This ROUTINE can be as basic or as complicated as your imagination will allow.

Standing in place "marking" the RHYTHMS, step out the following UNITS as you count the actual beats of music:

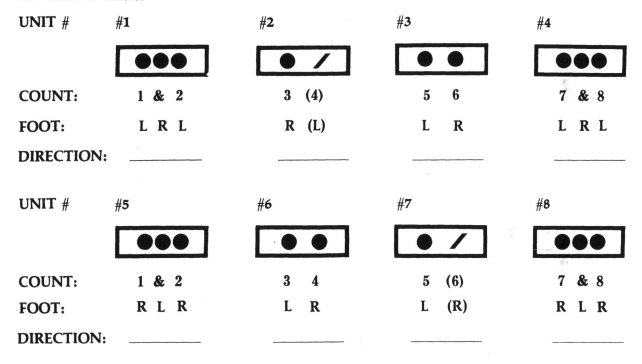

UNIT #	#1	#2	#3	#4
COUNT:	1 & 2	3 (4)	5 6	7 & 8
FOOT:	L R L	R (L)	L R	L R L
DIRECTION:	_____	_____	_____	_____

UNIT #	#5	#6	#7	#8
COUNT:	1 & 2	3 4	5 (6)	7 & 8
FOOT:	R L R	L R	L (R)	R L R
DIRECTION:	_____	_____	_____	_____

I have left out the "DIRECTION" because YOU are now the choreographer. If you do the RHYTHM PATTERN in place until it becomes comfortable, it will be easy to add DIRECTION.

> NOTE: •The second and 7th UNITS could be a "STEP KICK" or "STEP TOUCH"
> •Any of the TRIPLES could be a "SIDE TOGETHER SIDE"
> •The DOUBLE RHYTHM UNITS could be a "WALK WALK" or "SIDE TOGETHER"

These are just suggestions in case you don't know where to start. Use the above ROUTINE PHRASE to different kinds of music . . . and at different tempos. Done to MUSIC, this could be an interesting solo routine. For advanced students and teachers . . . this could be a four bar introduction to a SAMBA or CHA CHA routine.

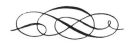

By count . . . the above routine would be referred to as TWO sets of EIGHT (meaning two sets of eight beats each) OR . . . an EIGHT UNIT ROUTINE. If you are really DOING the above routine to different kinds of music it should start being FUN . . . FAST . . . AND EASY! IS IT? Doing this routine to DISCO MUSIC will give you time to think of creative things to do with your hands and arms. More than the routine itself, concentrate on the COMPONENTS that go to make up the routine . . . THINK OF EACH INDIVIDUAL UNIT.

For ADVANCED MATERIAL, sometimes we "delay" a step . . . "syncopate" a step . . . or do a complete "stop" for a number of beats (which would be indicated by the use of a BLANK UNIT). NONE of these terms are important at this time except to point out that they exist and to emphasize that learning these three BASIC UNITS (adding direction, style and movement) will make you MORE than a competent dancer. YOU HAVE THE KEY to becoming as good as your efforts and determination will allow. . . .

The following questions are designed to make you THINK. DON'T LOOK BACK FOR THE ANSWERS UNTIL YOU'VE REALLY TRIED TO FIGURE THEM OUT. THE MORE YOU THINK FOR YOURSELF, THE SOONER THE "LANGUAGE" OF THE DANCE WILL BE YOURS.

1. If I do one SINGLE RHYTHM UNIT, one DOUBLE and one TRIPLE . . . how many beats of music will it take? _____

2. If I do a LEFT TRIPLE which foot will be free at the end of the unit? _____

3. A STEP FORWARD or BACKWARD is done in which foot position? _____

4. One UNIT "Marks time" . . . that means that whichever foot is free at the beginning of the unit . . . that SAME foot is STILL free at the END of the UNIT. Which RHYTHM UNIT "MARKS TIME?" _____

RECAP OF UNITS AND FOOT POSITIONS

PRIMARY UNITS

SECONDARY UNITS

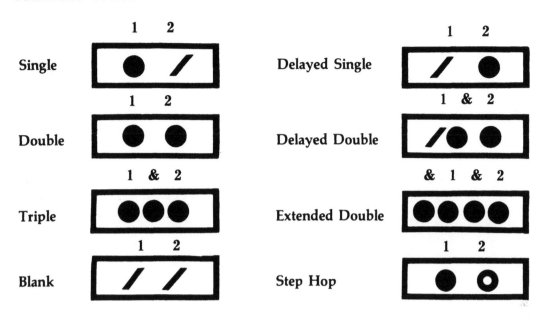

Single

Double

Triple

Blank

Delayed Single

Delayed Double

Extended Double

Step Hop

FOOT POSITIONS

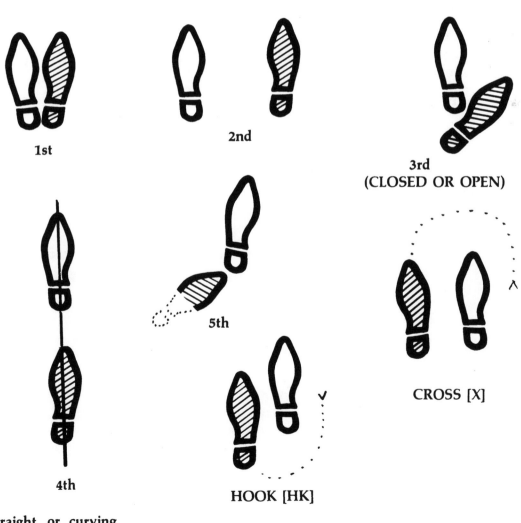

1st

2nd

3rd
(CLOSED OR OPEN)

4th

straight or curving
on any angle

5th

HOOK [HK]

CROSS [X]

19

CASE HISTORY:

A teacher from one of the JUNIOR COLLEGES reported the following experiment:

She had taught a BASIC SOCIAL DANCE CLASS for one Semester BEFORE being introduced to the UNIVERSAL UNIT SYSTEM. Then she attended DANCE CAMP to study for the three day TEACHERS SESSION covering the Universal Unit System.

Returning to school, she taught the INTERMEDIATE CLASS (second semester) using the system she had started with . . . But conducted the NEW BEGINNERS CLASS in the UNIT SYSTEM.

She then reports that at the end of that session, BOTH CLASSES WERE EQUAL. The FIRST SEMESTER CLASS had learned the material for both the BEGINNER AND THE INTERMEDIATE sessions.

(Teachers name and School on request) quoted with permission.

Jayne Unander, noted Cotillion teacher from Los Angeles, California refers to the UNITS as "POLKA DOT DANCING." The simplicity lies in stepping ONE TIME for each DOT . . . No DOT-No STEP . . . It's that easy.

Chapter III

MOVEMENT UNITS AND THEIR RELATIONSHIP TO THE DANCE. . .

We have said that a | UNIT | was | TWO BEATS OF MUSIC.

What is happening in the FEET (weight changes and direction) becomes the actual STEP PATTERN. The MOVEMENT (or lack of Movement) adds character, form and style to the Dance, and is recognized as a MOVEMENT UNIT.

When we refer to BASIC MOVEMENT UNITS we are referring to the actual Movement of the Center Point of Balance (CPB) within the framework of a TWO BEAT UNIT. The CPB is raised or lowered on a specific count.

Standing with the feet apart (2nd Foot Position) practice the following MOVEMENT UNITS to music. Swing or Disco Music with a Strong Bass Beat is best for practicing Movement.

If the MOVEMENT is UP on count ONE, it means that the CPB will reach its peak of rise on that specific count.

COUNT:	1	2		3	4		5	6		7	8
MOVEMENT UNIT:	UP	DOWN		UP	DOWN		UP	DOWN		UP	DOWN
Weight on:	LEFT	Foot		RIGHT	Foot		LEFT	Foot		RIGHT	Foot

Now listen to the music and REVERSE the MOVEMENT. (Listen for the Downbeat on ONE.)

COUNT:	1	2		3	4		5	6		7	8
MOVEMENT UNIT:	DOWN	UP		DOWN	UP		DOWN	UP		DOWN	UP
Weight on:	LEFT	Foot		RIGHT	Foot		LEFT	Foot		RIGHT	Foot

Now . . . DROP on every count, like a bouncing ball, alternating feet on every UNIT. Accent the DROP rather than the rise. Just like a bouncing ball, the ACTION is the ball going down to the floor. The REACTION is when it bounces back up. The ACTION of a Bouncing Unit is DOWN on count ONE and DOWN on count TWO. The "and" counts are the REACTION, or the lilting UP moves.

COUNT:	1	2		3	4		5	6		7	8
MOVEMENT UNIT:	DOWN	DOWN		DOWN	DOWN		DOWN	DOWN		DOWN	DOWN
Weight on:	LEFT	Foot		RIGHT	Foot		LEFT	Foot		RIGHT	Foot

The next MOVEMENT is a PRESS into the floor which produces an UP MOVEMENT on every count. This PRESSING of the Ball of the foot into the floor . . . is one of the most important elements in BODY MOVEMENT and CONTROL.

COUNT:	1	2		3	4		5	6		7	8
MOVEMENT UNIT:	UP	UP		UP	UP		UP	UP		UP	UP
Weight on:	LEFT	Foot		RIGHT	Foot		LEFT	Foot		RIGHT	Foot

All of these MOVEMENT UNITS have been VERTICAL MOVEMENT. Almost ALL Dance has some degree of VERTICAL MOVEMENT. Movement that SEEMS to be level, is almost always a VERTICAL MOVEMENT that has been S T R E T C H E D out until it appears as a HORIZONTAL MOVEMENT. The PRESS into the floor, freeing the toes, propels the CPB through space, producing HORIZONTAL MOVEMENT (Body Flight).

Practice these BASIC MOVEMENTS until you become familiar with the different variations and the body is able to respond to the music with any given MOVEMENT UNIT.

(TEACHERS NOTE: Have the student actually place his hand at the CPB to become aware of his CENTER and the movement that it produces.) It is the BODY that DANCES. The following exercise will clarify the difference between WALKING and DANCING.

THINK TALL! Place the hand at the CPB and lift up, as if you were pressing the top of your head on the ceiling. Now experiment by moving an arm or a leg in any direction. By adjusting your balance you will find that you can still stay in the same place.

Next . . . push the CPB in ANY direction . . . and you will find that you will have to transfer your weight to the other foot. The CPB is the KEY to all coordinated movement. PLACE the CPB in the spot where you wish to place your foot. The FOOT will receive the body . . . but the CPB moves FIRST.

To be IN TIME with the music . . . it is important that the actual weight transference take place on the beat. (The CPB completely transferred) and not just the act of the foot being placed on the floor.

To help develop the feeling of BODY FLIGHT . . . travel around the room counter-clockwise (LOD) doing SINGLE RHYTHM UNITS. The verbal call will be, "DRIVE brush, DRIVE brush." The soles of the feet act as a tire tread to propel the body forward. The FREE FOOT receives the body and continues the action forward.

To really understand MOVEMENT and to be able to control ALL PARTS of the body, it is necessary to isolate one's thinking into a specific area. The following HAND, ARM, HEAD and SHOULDER EXERCISES are good "Warm-Ups" for any class . . . and an excellent way to discipline the body for Dance. (YES . . . for SOCIAL DANCE also!)

TO THE MUSIC . . . Practice the BASIC MOVEMENT UNITS . . . Then add the following:

HEAD UNITS: (Rotate the head to the Left and to the Right on each count.)

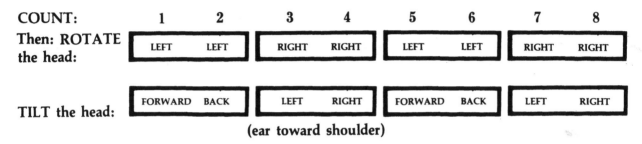

COUNT:	1	2	3	4	5	6	7	8
Then: ROTATE the head:	LEFT	LEFT	RIGHT	RIGHT	LEFT	LEFT	RIGHT	RIGHT

TILT the head:	FORWARD	BACK	LEFT	RIGHT	FORWARD	BACK	LEFT	RIGHT

(ear toward shoulder)

ROLL the head: (in a circle making a full roll for every unit.)

ARM UNITS: Do one arm at a time and then do both together.

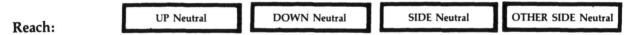

Reach:	UP Neutral	DOWN Neutral	SIDE Neutral	OTHER SIDE Neutral

A Chapter on MOVEMENT would not be complete without a discussion on FORCE POINT. While we are working on ARM MOVEMENTS, this is a good opportunity to see FORCE POINT in action.

1. Place your RIGHT hand in front of you . . . to the FAR LEFT.

2. Thinking into the HAND itself, place the FINGERTIPS to the extreme RIGHT on count ONE of the music (hold for two). The FORCE POINT has been the fingertips.

3. Now place the RIGHT hand to the FAR LEFT again and think into the ELBOW. FORCE the ELBOW to the far RIGHT and let the rest of the arm follow. The ELBOW has now become the FORCE POINT.

4. Repeat the same process (RIGHT hand to far LEFT) using the SHOULDER as the FORCE POINT and let the whole arm follow through. An entirely different effect has been created.

FORCE POINT becomes important when you realize how many times we are unable to decipher why one person looks "Sharp" while another looks "gnah!" doing what SEEMS to be the same moves. One looks controlled, coordinated . . . the other slightly awkward. When we know what to look for . . . it is easy to see the FORCE POINT in all movement.

Time to isolate the UPPER from the LOWER SPINE . . . and here are the exercises: (Again . . . do these to Music for better coordination training.)

There are TWO spots in the spine that can bend. We readily think of the spot at the waist. That is the easy one. The difficult one is centered between the shoulder blades. It is this UPPER SPINE flexibility that gives a Dancer that controlled but flexible look. It readily separates the Amateur from the Professional.

23

1. Think into the spine at the waistline. Lean BACK, bending at the waistline. You will find it difficult to breathe and there will be a strain at the neck. If you were to dance in this position, you would have a bad back in very short order.

2. Now think up into the center of the shoulder blades. We have to FIND those muscles before we can control them. As you think of tilting the body back from that particular spot, you will find that it RELEASES the lung area and makes breathing easier. The shoulders are free to sway in any direction. The TOP of the body feels centered in the CPB and you are on your way to total flexibility.

3. Thinking into your CENTER (CPB) push to the RIGHT and to the LEFT. Alternate directions to music and gradually build up your flexibility.

4. Give the LOWER SPINE a workout by using the HIPS as a FORCE POINT. Keep the upper part of the body very still and move the hips on every count.

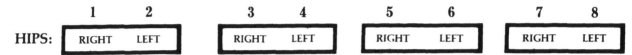

	1	2		3	4		5	6		7	8
HIPS:	RIGHT	LEFT		RIGHT	LEFT		RIGHT	LEFT		RIGHT	LEFT

(Next try hitting the same side twice and alternate sides.)

With the feet together (1st Foot Position) release the heels and let the heels swing WITH the hip movement. (See BODY LANGUAGE.)

SHOULDERS: . . .

How we control the shoulders, carrying them at ease, or emphasizing with a sharp move, adds much to the Dance. Practice these exercises noting the DIFFERENCE between one move and another . . . BOTH have the same LOOK to an untrained eye.

PUSH the RIGHT Shoulder Forward on every count . . . 1 2 3 4 5 6 7 8

Now, PULL the LEFT shoulder Back on every count . . . 1 2 3 4 5 6 7 8

If someone were to take a PICTURE of the above moves, they might look the same. However, the feeling and the ACTUAL LOOK of the move are different.

Practice reversing the above:

PUSH the LEFT Shoulder Forward on every count . . . 1 2 3 4 5 6 7 8

Now, PULL the RIGHT Shoulder Back on every count . . . 1 2 3 4 5 6 7 8

(Note the importance of these exercises for the Lady in New York Hustle.)

Advanced MOVES in the Legs would include POPS and BRACES.

Put both feet together in 1st foot position and picture a DRUM in front of your knees. A "POP" is a sharp move as if both knees would HIT the drum on a specific beat. Try POPS to a count of 8. (This particular move was popular during the Freestyle ROCK period, but is still important for contrast to other moves.)

BRACES consist of BRACING the knees BACK one every count. If the HEELS are released, the action will make you travel backward. This exercise is necessary to perform the "Goin Nowhere" which resembles a man riding a bike . . . in one place.

BRACE Both knees back on every count.

BRACE ONE knee back with the other bent on count ONE (hold two).

BRACE the OTHER knee back on count THREE (hold four).

(The body will travel slightly back each time.)

Eventually you will be able to BRACE back on EVERY COUNT, alternating feet (used in Swing or Disco Freestyle).

BREATHING

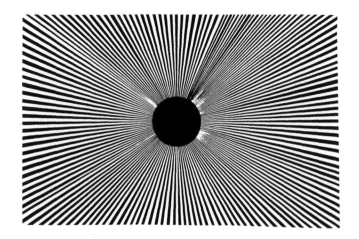

BREATHING is something that we all assume we MUST be doing . . . or we just wouldn't be alive. Well we ARE all breathing . . . but the average person uses such a small part of the lung capacity that it is a wonder that we have any energy at all. In YOGA, breathing exercises are emphasized to "clear the lungs" of stale air . . . to renew strength and energy . . . and to develop a RHYTHM in movement. How does this affect our DANCING? Try this exercise and see if you can tell the difference. (This is PARTICULARLY VALUABLE to COMPETITION DANCERS and PERFORMERS. . . .)

• Lift the RIB CAGE . . . Press the top of the head toward the ceiling . . . exhale every bit of breath that you can squeeze out. Then inhale very slowly.

• Now . . . Put on some music. (Whatever turns you on . . . Disco to Tango to Ballet!!) Now . . . DANCING to the music . . . Breathe IN for a full measure of music.

• 1. Breathe IN for a full FOUR COUNTS of MUSIC (one full measure of 4/4 time).

• 2. Breathe OUT for FOUR COUNTS of MUSIC.

• 3. Continue to dance, breathing slowly and deeply in time with the music.

If the MUSIC is 4/4 time . . . Keep the measured breathing at 4 counts IN and 4 counts OUT. If you are dancing to WALTZ MUSIC . . . change to 3 counts IN and 3 counts OUT.

Practice will reward you well with increased endurance . . . a feeling of buoyancy . . . and a feeling of a deeper connection with the MUSIC.

• When you become proficient in your breathing, you will be able to BREATHE IN for a FULL EIGHT COUNTS . . . and breathe OUT for a FULL EIGHT COUNTS. You will be amazed at the increase in energy and endurance.*

*Thruout the writing of this book, the breathing exercises, as simply done as they are explained above, kept up the energy level thru many "all nite" work sessions. They can help more than just in the Dance.

The study of Movement to Music should make you more aware of all of the individual parts of the body. Getting those individual PARTS to respond one at a time . . . will lead to being able to control ALL of the parts at the same time.

Students of YOGA will relate to these exercises in that the principal is the same. Each is working toward the development and control of the whole being. Learn first to be AWARE of each part . . . Then to move and CONTROL each part . . . Then free the parts and let them respond to the music on their own.

You're going to be a GREAT Dancer!!

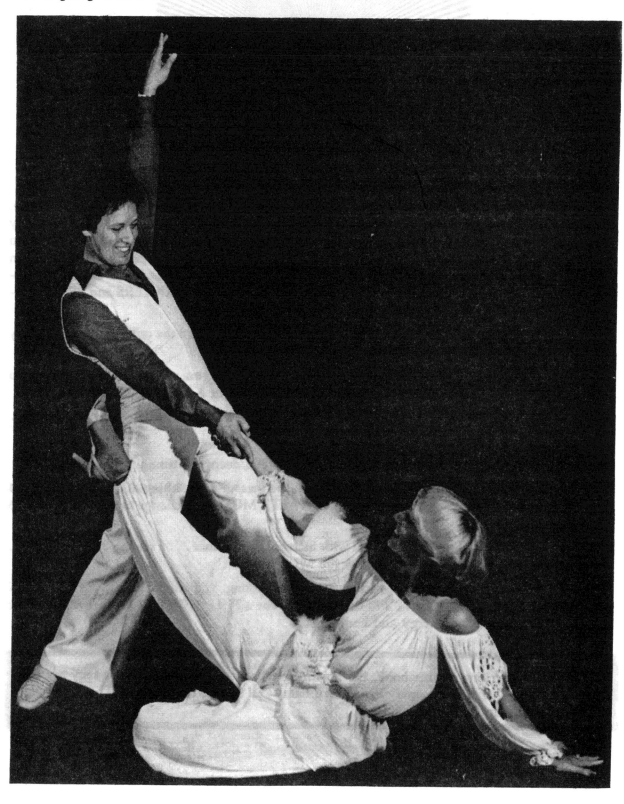

Golden State Dance Teachers Association

Reprint from TEACHERS TRAINING at

SQUAW VALLEY DANCE CAMP — 1974.

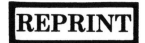

Some Basic Exercises to establish the RHYTHMS and the VARIETY of FOOT PLACEMENTS that are possible. START with these and then make up your own.

1 2	1 2	1 and 2
SINGLE RHYTHM	DOUBLE RHYTHM	TRIPLE RHYTHM

SINGLE RHYTHM

"Step Touch"
2nd to 1st
4th to 1st
4th to 3rd

"Step Point"
1st to 2nd
1st to 4th
2nd to 5th
4th to 4th

"Step Kick"
2nd — X Fwd.
1st — Side

"Step Stamp"
2nd to 4th

DOUBLE RHYTHM

"Step Step"
4th to 4th
Fwd. Fwd.
Fwd. Bk.
Bk. Fwd.
Bk. Bk.

"Side Together"
2nd to 1st

"Side Cross"
2nd to X

"Walk Hook"
4th to Hook

"Fwd. Side"
4th to 2nd

TRIPLE RHYTHM

"Step Step Step"

"Side Together Side"
2nd   1st   2nd

"Run Run Run"
4th   4th   4th

"Bk.   Tog.   Fwd."
4th   1st   4th

"Check and Strike"
4th   4th   1st

"Hook Triple"
5th   2nd   5th
(Half turn)

"Fwd.   Tog.   Back"
4th   1st   4th

DELAYED SINGLE:

(corresponds to Chain Studio concept of "double rhythm" ("tap step" in Swing).

For many years RHYTHM CHANGES have been taught . . . particularly in Swing, but also in the Latin dances.. However, it was not a COMPLETE system in that it only related to a PORTION of the pattern and only specific dances. The Skippy Blair UNIT SYSTEM (copyright 1963) included EIGHT BASIC UNITS, out of which ALL Patterns in ALL the ballroom dances were composed. The text book "So You Want To Learn To Dance" used that system and the system gained in popularity thru the years. It DID take concentrated effort to learn and so was limited in its scope. TEN YEARS later with constant work on SYSTEM . . . METHOD . . . CONTINUITY . . .RELEVANCE . . . etc., the NEW UNIT SYSTEM boils down to only THREE BASIC UNITS and is understandable immediately. MODERN JAZZ and the current ROCK VARIATIONS are easily choreographed, starting with the BASIC RHYTHM UNITS . . . adding the MOVEMENT UNITS . . . and then putting them in sequence.

Chapter IV
YOUR DANCING IMAGE

First . . . Remember that we are ALWAYS conveying a picture of what we are. When we TALK, we have the opportunity to explain WHO we are, how we FEEL etc. When we DANCE, we project an image in MIME. "MIME" is communication without words.

What IMAGE does your dancing project? In specific dances, the image should be one that conveys the FEELING of the dance, and still have the essence of YOU in the dance.

With so much emphasis on BODY LANGUAGE today, it pays to be aware of the image we wish to project. Always THINK "UP." Even in the dances that settle in the knees, the C.P.B. (Center Point of Balance) should be lifted with an elegance that tells the world that you are a worthwhile individual. It is also easier to breathe and less tiring.

FOOTWORK is also important in the projection of the overall image:

TOE OUT too far and you resemble CHARLIE CHAPLIN. It takes on a comical look and throws the body out of line.

TOE IN and the look is one of WEAKNESS or STUPIDITY. (Character actors will "toe in" to add authenticity to a WEAK CHARACTER).

CLASSIC FOOTWORK is best achieved by adhering to the BASIC FOOT POSITIONS (See Chapter I). Practice walking a straight line in FOURTH FOOT POSITION. Note that the center of your HEEL and the center of your BIG TOE should be on the same line.

Check your shoes to see that the soles are worn evenly. If they are worn down on the OUTSIDE of the foot, your weight is rolling to the outside and will produce a club footed look. It also has an unsteady "feel" and can be corrected by gaining CONTROL of the entire foot. Loose feet project an awkward image.

For girls in particular, BACKWARD STEPS can project an awkward look. Make sure that one foot goes directly behind the other. "DOUBLE TRACKING," with the feet APART is only for COMEDY ROLES. Keep the shoulders UP and carefully place one foot behind the other as you travel backward. Think of ONE STRAIGHT LINE and STEP ON IT.

ARM MOVEMENTS should enhance the dance by adding LINE and SYMMETRY. Exaggerated arms are for performance, and even then should be used with caution. Determine the DESIRED PICTURE. Look in a mirror. What does your IMAGE SAY?

In each dance, study carefully the MOOD of the dance and the GENERAL CHARACTERISTICS of the dance. Try not to let one style dominate and carry over into all of the other dances. (We all know people who "WALTZ" their Foxtrot, or who SWING their Cha Cha). Dancing is far more fun when the FEELINGS of the dance are separated and interpreted.

PROJECT HAPPINESS: . . . Smile when you dance. Laugh if the opportunity presents itself. Don't be afraid to ENJOY the dance. Nothing destroys the dance so much as someone looking as though the whole thing was either HARD WORK . . . or, worse yet, BORING.

PROJECT CONFIDENCE . . . Know your patterns so well that variations flow with ease. Dance only the material that you can dance with confidence. Save the NEW MATERIAL and the HARD MATERIAL for practice sessions.

Remember that we are TALKING, NON-VERBALLY when we dance. We tell more about ourselves than we realize. Further than that, we can BECOME that which we project, by first FEELING the part, and then projecting THAT IMAGE in the dance.

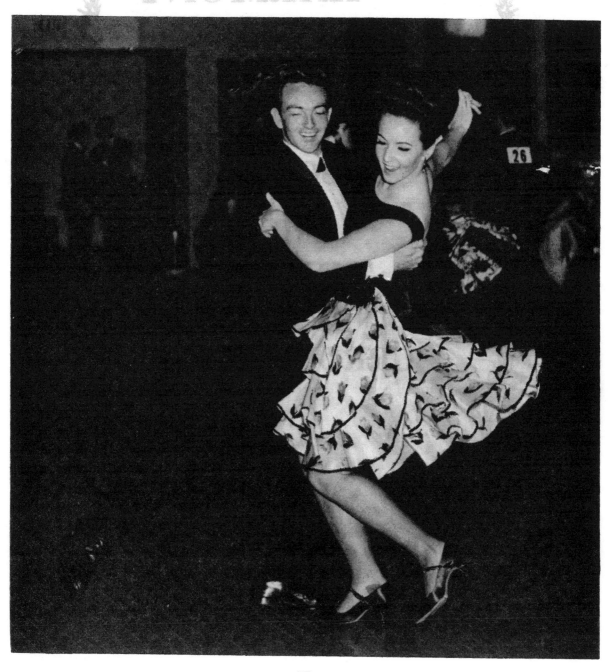

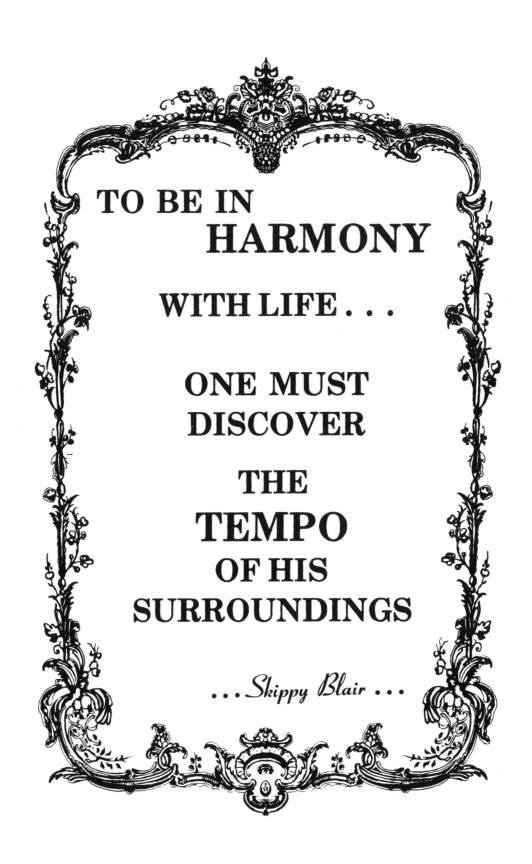

TO BE IN
HARMONY

WITH LIFE . . .

ONE MUST
DISCOVER

THE

TEMPO
OF HIS
SURROUNDINGS

. . . *Skippy Blair* . . .

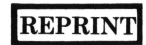

Whether you are entering a local NITECLUB COMPETITION or you have worked your way thru endless Preliminaries and are part of a NATIONAL FINAL, the following thoughts might be important. (Based on more than 20 years training Contestants.)

It may sound trite to say that it doesn't matter who wins or loses . . . that it is HOW WE PLAYED THE GAME THAT COUNTS. Trite or not . . . It really is true. There has NEVER been a Competition that did not leave MANY PEOPLE UNHAPPY. A Dance Competition is not like a foot race where one crosses the line before another. It is a matter of PREFERENCE by a number of Judges who may or may not agree with your own evaluation of what it takes to win first place.

Entering a Competition gives you a CHANCE TO BE SEEN. If you are entering ONLY TO WIN, do yourself a favour and DON'T ENTER. A Competition should give you a REASON to better your craft. It should give you a DEADLINE to work toward, so that an end is in sight. It should give you the opportunity to perform in front of your Peers . . . for their approval and YOUR satisfaction. The judging itself is dependent on too many variables. The OUTCOME of the Competition should be the LEAST important factor.

Part of the Game of participation is being able to DANCE YOUR VERY BEST and be CONTENT with that. A "WELL DONE" from a trusted friend is more important to me than FIRST PLACE. Just BEING IN A COMPETITION gives you the prestige of BEING SOMEONE. You get to be known for your CAPABILITIES and for your GROWTH. You will also be known for your SPORTSMANSHIP. Competition is NOT A CHILD'S GAME. Before entering, resolve to BE AN ADULT . . . WIN . . . LOSE . . . OR DRAW!!

In evaluating some of the recent HUSTLE COMPETITIONS (only those of STATEWIDE or NATIONAL significance) I have found that the same rules apply no matter WHAT dance is being done. When the RULES of the Competition come up with the BEST DANCERS as their WINNERS, then you know that you have to better your Craft in order to compete.

Observing the BIG FINALS at DILLONS in Los Angeles in May of '78, all of the varieties of styles and form were in evidence. Fortunately the FIRST PLACE went to the most obvious BEST DANCERS in the contest. The INTERESTING part was that any number of the other couples COULD have been first. In each case, the other couples made the usual errors that separate the AMATEUR from the PROFESSIONAL. A Competition is a SHOW. It must be CHOREOGRAPHED in order to understand and develop the various highlites of the number.

As chairman* of judges of the $10,000.00 series of Competitions at the CRESCENDO, (Anaheim, Cal.) it is my privilege to see many really fine dancers in various stages of development. It is gratifying to have these contestants come back and show you the improvements they have made because of the comments that had been written on their judging sheet. Repeatedly, these contestants, as well as those from Dillons . . . and almost every other contest observed, displayed these same problem areas. . . .

Too many of the couples had small segments choreographed and relied on JUST DANCING in between. Most of the errors came in an attempt at TWO STEP. TWO STEP is fascinating to do and fun to watch when it is done PROPERLY. However, without knowing EXACTLY when you are going to change from one dance to another, the lady is at the mercy of her partner. When the chips are down and there are two couples with equal talent, the couple who UNDERSTANDS every move they make will look more CONFIDENT and more POLISHED. Today's Dancers are becoming more and more knowledgeable. If you wish to compete, learn your craft. Find yourself a good Dance Coach and then LISTEN to the advice that is given. It is very difficult to see yourself as others see you. Don't be satisfied with getting by. Resolve to rise to your OWN HIGHEST POTENTIAL . . . because that's what LIFE IS REALLY ALL ABOUT!!! (And GOOD LUCK in your next Competition.)

G.S.D.T.A. CONTEST WINNERS
1958 thru 1978

G.S.D.T.A. has produced some notable COMPETITION DANCERS as well as PER-FORMERS and TEACHING SPECIALISTS. Some of the HIGHLITES include:

1958 . . . Bob Trageser and Carlene Rose . . . (pictured with Al and Marilyn Jarvis and Skippy Blair) Winners of the first $500.00 JARVIS SHOW FINAL.

1962 . . . John Buckner and Merilou Puopolo (Miss Downey 1961, Miss L.A. 1963) Many time winners on the Let's Dance T.V. show.

1964 . . . Mike Mikita and Pat "Lucky" Armstrong, winners of the California Junior Dance Championship for D.E.A. and FIRST PLACE winners the same year at the NEW YORK WORLD'S FAIR.

1965 . . . Corky Elser and Andrea Lee (now Kluge) performers and contest winners together, and with numerous other partners.

1966 . . . Corky Elser and Sheila Blair, California Professional Champions in Latin and Swing.

1974 . . . Larry Kern and Sheila Blair, following a successful season in Las Vegas as headliners . . . won several Swing competitions.

1958

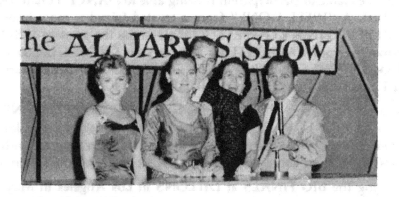

1962

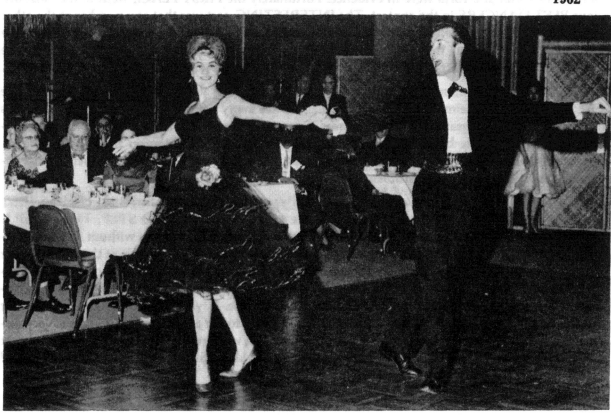

32

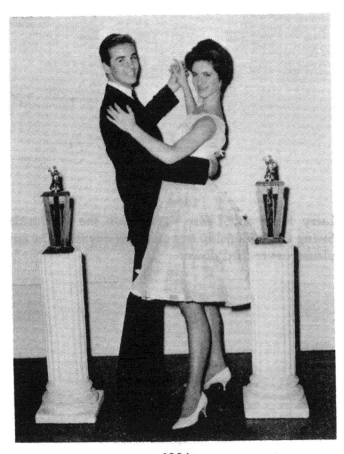

1964

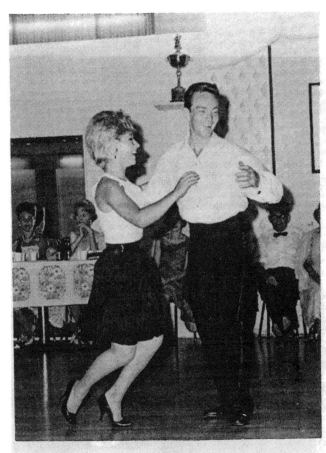

1965

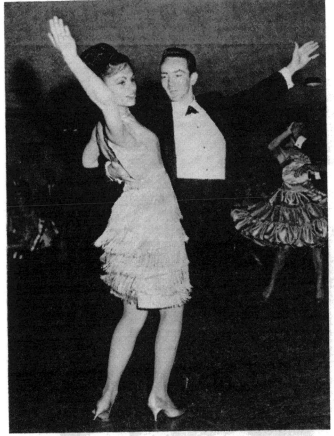

1966

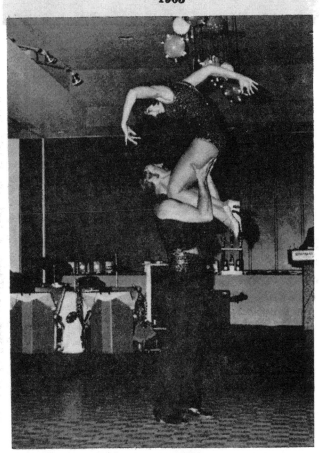

1974

33

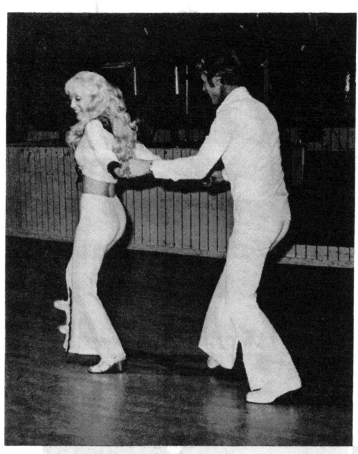

1975 . . .
Larry Kern and Lynn Vogen won the California
Swing Championship to a standing ovation. The ap-
plause never died down.

1978 . . .
Buddy Schwimmer and Lynn Vogen topped the
Southern California scene by winning a spot on the
Merv Griffin Show . . . and then placed second in the
whole country.

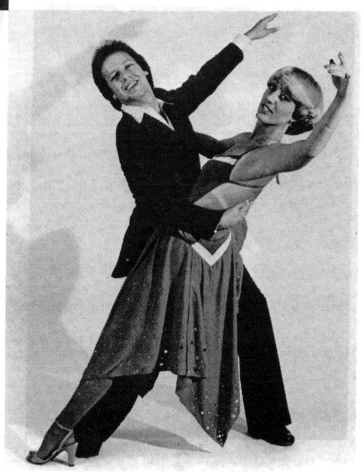

Chapter V

THE ESSENCE OF CONTEMPORARY DANCE

The ESSENCE of a particular dance is the "FEELING" or "LOOK" that sets it apart from all other dances. Recognizing the DIFFERENCES, rather than the SIMILARITIES to existing dances, is what makes a knowledgable CONTEMPORARY DANCER.

Many CONTEMPORARY DANCES are mistaken for certain existing dances because of similar characteristics. Let's explore those SIMILARITIES in order to understand the ESSENCE of each unique dance.

For starters, the popular TWO STEP is often confused with SAMBA. SAMBA is a FUN DANCE and is compatible with much of the Contemporary Music. However, SAMBA is NOT TWO STEP. When the two dances are combined, confusion sets in. Dancing EITHER dance is exciting and fun as long as you KNOW which you are doing and are able to isolate the differences.

The SIMILARITIES are many. BOTH dances are composed of two TRIPLE RHYTHM UNITS. BOTH dances are FOUR BEATS of music for a Basic Step. The MOVEMENT is VERTICAL and the subtle BOUNCE is recognizable as a CHARACTERISTIC of BOTH DANCES.

Now to the DIFFERENCES, and therein lies the KEY to good dancing. The VERTICAL RHYTHM in SAMBA (subtle as it may be) is DOWN and DOWN. That is: the BODY MOVEMENT actually settles on count ONE and on count TWO. The rise or PRESS is on the "AND" count before the ONE. This produces what we call a subtle BOUNCE. (SUBTLE because it is felt more than seen.)

The MOVEMENT UNIT for TWO STEP is the OPPOSITE. The subtle VERTICAL RHYTHM is UP on count ONE and also UP on count TWO. This produces a MOVEMENT UNIT of UP UP. It is achieved by pressing the ball of the foot into the floor on every count.

Another IMPORTANT difference is the actual placement of foot positions in the individual dances. Although both dances are composed of TWO TRIPLE RHYTHM UNITS, the foot placement is quite different:

TWO STEP: The accent is BACK on count ONE of the UNIT and SIDE on count TWO. The ONE becomes a ROCK BACK in a sort of SPRING ACTION.

SAMBA HUSTLE: (Samba patterns to Contemporary Music). The accent is FORWARD or BACK or SIDE on count ONE and STAYS on that step until the very last second before continuing the rest of the pattern. There is NO ROCKING STEP.

35

TWO STEP			SAMBA HUSTLE (or Samba)		
COUNT:	1 and 2		1 and a 2		
UNIT:	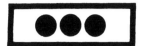		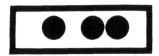		
DIRECTION:	B Fpl S		S 5th Fpl		
MOVEMENT:	Up Up		Down Down		
FOOTWORK:	Toe Flat Flat		Flat & Toe Flat		
RESISTANCE:	Away		With		

Viewing the DIFFERENCE between one dance and the other, it becomes apparent why MIXING the two would be almost impossible. The body would be incapable of transmitting the change of movement and style from one pattern to the next. (See chapter on Competition Dancing.)

However, MOST of the Contemporary Dances can be danced to the same music. Some fits better than others, but the fascinating part of today's music is the VARIETY of RHYTHM INSTRUMENTS which allows a VARIETY of INTERPRETATION.

HOW THEN do we MIX the various dances without MIXING THEM UP? We MIX by inserting RHYTHM BREAKS between one form of dance and another. For instance . . .

4 UNITS of TWO STEP followed by a RHYTHM BREAK of 2 UNITS of PIVOTS.

Follow that with 4 UNITS of Contemporary FOXTROT and you are ready to REPEAT the process or add another RHYTHM BREAK . . . like 2 UNITS of SALSA VALIENTE (FOUR SHORT WALKING STEPS, stepping on every beat). Use those walking steps to put the girl in OPEN POSITION and you would be ready to do a few patterns in NEWPORTER SALSA.

Never move from one FORM of TRIPLE to ANOTHER FORM of TRIPLE without inserting a series of RHYTHM BREAKS. RHYTHM BREAKS consist mostly of DOUBLE RHYTHM variations that can be done in any dance. The STYLE or MOVEMENT may vary, but the actual pattern remains the same.

RHYTHM BREAKS

1. a series of PIVOTS (either Left or Right)
2. CHASSES or GRAPEVINES (all DOUBLE RHYTHM)
3. a POSE or DROP or LIFT that "HOLDS" for at least 2 counts
   (can take as much as two, three or four UNITS)
4. a series of short WALKING STEPS as in SALSA VALIENTE

NEW YORK HUSTLE ? . . . LATIN HUSTLE ?
. . . CALIFORNIA SHUFFLE ? . . . GOLDEN STATE SWING ?

Again, for the purpose of IDENTIFICATION, you will find that all of the MYSTERY has been taken out of the various dances, by isolating the various FORMS so that teaching becomes a pleasure. It is impossible to teach 20 different FORMS of HUSTLE. Having researched all areas . . . and numerous teachers . . . and hundreds of just plain good dancers, it becomes easy to isolate THREE MAIN FORMS:

1. The LINE HUSTLE where all are doing the same things.

2. The SAME FOOT HUSTLE where BOTH PARTNERS start on the same foot but are dancing as a couple. (started in California and is just now hitting New York and other areas across the country). Called here: LATIN HUSTLE.

3. The OPPOSITE FOOT HUSTLE . . . done as a couple. It is this OPPOSITE FOOT HUSTLE that has so many different names . . . even though the PATTERNS are the SAME but with VARYING RHYTHMS. The STRUCTURE is the same. They are all THREE UNIT PATTERNS . . . (6 beats of music). They all have the same ESSENCE and ATTITUDE. Here in California we have weeded out the various names, (NEW YORK HUSTLE, SPANISH HUSTLE, LATIN HUSTLE). In that the STRUCTURE is the same, we identify all of those dances under one name . . . "NEW YORK HUSTLE." All three RHYTHM variations are used from time to time but the MAIN RHYTHM PATTERN is: DELAYED SINGLE/ TRIPLE/ DOUBLE . . . The VERBAL PATTERN is TAP STEP/ STEP THREE TIMES/ and STEP STEP. The count is: 1 2/ 3&4/ 5 6/.

4. THE CALIFORNIA SHUFFLE refers to the SYNCOPATION that is a series of: STEP POINT, STEP POINT, STEP POINT, STEP POINT etc. The "POINTS" are on the actual count. The STEPS are on the "and" count. These can be done replacing the TRIPLES in SWING . . . or can be done BY THEMSELVES as a FREE FORM. They can be done IN PLACE or traveling in any direction. Another example of a RHYTHM PATTERN that has acquired a NAME of its own.

5. GOLDEN STATE SWING is the name given the G.S.D.T.A. specialized form of WEST COAST SWING. There are many stylings and specific patterns that are peculiar to G.S.D.T.A. that we thought it necessary to differentiate between just WEST COAST SWING and our particular version of the same dance.

The same IDENTITY PROBLEM exists with SALSA versus CHA CHA or MAMBO. The SIMILARITIES confuse the issue, but the ESSENCE separates the CONTEMPORARY DANCER from the dancer who "converts" an old standard to fit todays music.

6. SALSA PICADO: (The TRIPLES that look like MAMBO to the untrained eye). SALSA PICADO is the name coined for the little TRIPLE RHYTHM STEPS that have the characteristic of little "BREAKS" similar to those in MAMBO. The DIFFERENCE is in the MOVEMENT and the COUNT.

SALSA PICADO movement is a sublte DOWN on count ONE and UP on count TWO (a VERTICAL MOVEMENT). MAMBO is a HORIZONTAL MOVEMENT of the body as it projects FORWARD and BACKWARD. SALSA PICADO is TRIPLE RHYTHM which takes TWO UNITS or FOUR BEATS to complete a Basic Pattern. MAMBO is a FOUR UNIT PATTERN which takes EIGHT BEATS of music to complete a Basic Pattern. MAMBO can be danced to SALSA MUSIC by doubling the timing. It is INTERESTING. It is FUN . . . but it does not have the ESSENCE of the SALSA.

	SALSA PICADO				MAMBO					(Inverted
COUNT:	1 and 2				2	3		4	5	UNITS)
UNIT:	●●●				● ●			●		
DIRECTION:	T F Bpl				F	B		T		
MOVEMENT:	Down Up				Fwd.	Back				
FOOTWORK:	Flat Toe Flat				Toe	Flat		Flat		

(Note the difference between SALSA PICADO and SAMBA and TWO STEP. It is not that one is any better than another . . . only that we can RECOGNIZE and EXECUTE the difference.)

7. SALSA VALIENTE is merely a series of MARCHING STEPS that look very similar to PASO DOBLE' and sometimes MERENGUE. The ESSENCE of SALSA VALIENTE is the CLIMB and the ATTITUDE. The CLIMB refers to the BASIC MOVEMENT which spans TWO UNITS. The MOVEMENT lowers on count ONE and gradually rises through count FOUR. The ATTITUDE is that of most of the current SOCIAL DANCE ... one of CLASS ... of DIGNITY ... that look that says, "I AM SOMEBODY!" The patterns are simple in their construction in that there is a constant MARCHING of DOUBLE RHYTHM UNITS. The STYLE is the continuous use of ROPE ARMS. Many of the patterns are merely rearrangements of patterns from LATIN HUSTLE and other Contemporary Dances.

(See Chapter on SALSA for complete analysis of the Dance. Note definitions of TOE, FLAT, etc. in Chapter on TERMINOLOGY. Abbreviations listed under TERMINOLOGY.)

Another IDENTITY PROBLEM exists with DISCO SWING ... LINDY HUSTLE ... and SALSA.

8. DISCO SWING or LINDY HUSTLE ... In a recent publication (May 1978) a popular Choreographer printed breakdowns for this dance that turned out to be nothing more than the old BASIC BREAKDOWN for EASTERN SWING. This is a bit unfair to the dancing public. While EASTERN SWING may be fun to do to Contemporary Music, it bears little resemblance to its Contemporary Counterpart. To the untrained eye, what APPEARS to be a half-time EASTERN SWING is actually an entirely new Dance.

9. EASTERN SWING refers to the style of SWING where BOTH partners do a ROCK STEP away from each other, with the resistance on the BACK ROCK. It generally travels in a circular pattern. This is also a CHARACTERISTIC of the dance it resembles.

The DIFFERENCE is what makes the dance. The EASTERN SWING Basic RHYTHM PATTERN is a THREE UNIT PATTERN. (6 beats of music.) The ROCK STEP occurs on the DOUBLE RHYTHM UNIT (The "STEP STEP"). In the CONTEMPORARY DANCE, the ROCK STEP occurs in the TRIPLE RHYTHM UNIT on the "and" count. The DOUBLE RHYTHM UNITS all WALK FORWARD which is the exact opposite of the EASTERN SWING.

In trying to place this particular CONTEMPORARY DANCE, (which incidentally is VERY popular and in much use), we isolated the individual UNITS to compare the similarities and the differences to the better known dances. The RESULT WAS THIS:

A. The TRIPLE RHYTHM UNITS are identical to those of SALSA PICADO and the DOUBLE RHYTHM UNITS are walking steps (comparable to those in SALSA VALIENTE). Therefore, we have placed the Dance in the SALSA Category, with the SYNONYM of DISCO SWING because of the many UNDERARM TURNS.

B. Another important factor in this Dance is that, unlike any other form of SWING, the WALKING STEPS alternate the STARTING FOOT. The Man first walks in starting LEFT RIGHT. His next WALKING STEP starts RIGHT LEFT. (Lady does the natural opposite.) (see Chapter on SALSA for this Dance, under NEWPORTER SALSA.)

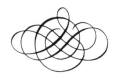

Golden State Dance Teachers Association

Note to Teachers, July 15, 1978

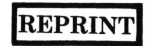

COMPARISON NEW YORK HUSTLE TO STREET HUSTLE

One Dance can evolve to become something better, more complicated, more stylish, more technical than in its basic form or creation. That is the natural order of things. Growth is ever present. However, if the evolvement becomes so changed in its growth that the ESSENCE becomes SOMETHING ELSE, it becomes another dance.

CHA CHA is an evolvement of MAMBO. First came Mambo. It was too complicated for the average dancer and was confined to the better dancers and teachers of dance.

Then came Triple Mambo to a little slower tempo. Finally CHA CHA came into existence. The FORM had changed to include an entirely different ESSENCE. It was a NEW DANCE.

NEW YORK HUSTLE (and all of its various RHYTHM COMBINATIONS . . . Spanish Hustle, American Hustle, Latin Hustle, etc.) is composed of THREE UNIT PATTERNS with a certain IDENTIFIABLE ESSENCE that says, "THIS IS NEW YORK HUSTLE!" . . . Then along came syncopations, which are an important evolvement of EVERY DANCE. (See basic syncopations of NEW YORK HUSTLE.) Some dancers saw these syncopations and also saw the quick weight changes involved in TWO STEP and confused one with the other. The result was what is commonly called STREET HUSTLE. The RHYTHM STRUCTURE is comparable to NEW YORK HUSTLE but the ESSENCE is entirely different.

We refer to STREET DANCING as those forms which evolve from a number of untrained dancers dancing what they THINK they see other people doing. If it is repeated enough times it takes on a character of its own . . . and becomes its own dance. (MOST important changes in Social Dance are as a result of STREET DANCING.)

The work of a CONTEMPORARY DANCE ANALYST is to dissect the various forms . . . and to be able to put themselves in the shoes of the STREET DANCER. By doing so, you can SEE what they see. You can also then dissect what they were TRYING to do . . . and come up with teachable, logical dance forms that have enough character to stand on their own, complete with BASIC PATTERNS up through advanced patterns that still maintain the ESSENCE or CHARACTER of the dance itself.

If you do a BOX STEP in FOXTROT and keep increasing the tempo . . . at some point you will be doing a BALBOA BASIC. However, at the point at which the CHARACTER CHANGES and one starts LOOKING LIKE BALBOA instead of FOXTROT, it has BECOME another dance. The ESSENCE has changed. In THIS INSTANCE the change has been brought about by TEMPO.

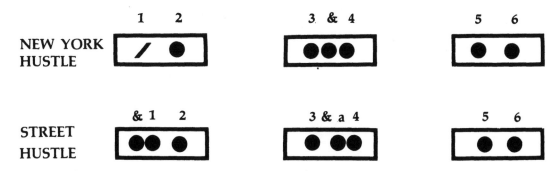

BLAIR ON "SATURDAY NIGHT FEVER"

(Reprint of Newspaper Article — April, 1978)

The year 1978 will go down in the History of Social Dance as the year of "Saturday Night Fever." Through the years, there have been many changes in Social Dancing ... the FAD dances of the era echo the MUSIC of the day. It is always the MUSIC that comes first ... and the dancers interpret the music. From a SOCIOLOGICAL point of view, the "Look" of the late 70's dancing is a healthy one. The ROCK era was an introverted, isolation type of dancing that allowed two people to dance as a couple without ever touching each other ... or, in many cases, without even LOOKING at each other. It was an era of non-involvement.

The NEW look is one of pride ... an upright posture with the head held high. The rib cage is lifted and an ATTITUDE of confidence permeates the scene. Dancing with a partner has become more important than dancing alone. The DRESS has become more formal and once more DANCING has become associated with DRESSING UP and LOOKING GOOD.

The current DANCE SCENE is a dancer's delight. The styles vary from VERY SIMPLE to EXTREMELY COMPLICATED ... and all points in between. It seems that all of the dances of yesterday have combined with the music of today and produced a contagious FEELING of Dance that encompasses unlimited variations in both PATTERN and STYLE.

From the standpoint of a STUDENT of DANCE, this is probably the most exciting dance era since the early 40's. Today, EVERYONE dances ... and the gap between BALLROOM STYLE AND NITECLUB style is closing fast. Contemporary dance is no longer the private property of the YOUTH of the day. All ages are getting caught up in the "Saturday Night Fever."

From a HISTORICAL point of view of dance, one sees the merging of age groups as an era of closer understanding ... the closing of the GENERATION GAP.

This era will be known for the merging of ideas. Houses and apartments done by top decorators include antiques along with contemporary pieces and achieve a feeling of good taste ... a blending of past and future. We see it in CLOTHES, in MUSIC, in FURNISHINGS ... and so it should be no surprise that it is also taking place in the dance.

It is important to note that although the STYLE changes, the UNIT STRUCTURE of contemporary dance has varied very little through the years. The early 70's saw the introduction out of New York of the HUSTLE and gradually various forms emerged across the country. LINE DANCES were first dubbed HUSTLE and then came LATIN HUSTLE, NEW YORK HUSTLE, and the SPANISH HUSTLE which are COUPLE DANCES. From that beginning followed the TANGO HUSTLE, CHA CHA HUSTLE, FOXTROT HUSTLE and so on ... covering the broad spectrum of all social dance. The LINE DANCES which had started to lose their popularity gained new strength with the showing of JOHN TRAVOLTA in SATURDAY NIGHT FEVER. The true blend had taken place.

The question is always before us ... WHO starts the new dances? And there is always someone ready to accept responsibility for its creation. The truth of the matter is that MANY people are starting the SAME DANCE at the SAME TIME all over the world ... because dancers react to MUSIC through FEELING. There may be slight differences, but the ESSENCE will be the same.

Chapter VI
DISCO-FREESTYLE

In ALL FREESTYLE DANCING (whether the BUS STOP . . . the SKEETER . . . HAND JIVE . . . or GET UP GET DOWN) whatever new "BIT" comes up tomorrow, one fact is certain . . .

They are ALL bits and pieces . . . arrangement and rearrangement of varying RHYTHM UNITS. Rather than DATE the material in this book, we have developed exercises, using all POSSIBLE combinations of these RHYTHM UNITS. That NEW DANCE that you will see TOMORROW, is already printed in this text. YOU are the explorer.

Arrange . . . and rearrange and you will not only discover EVERY DANCE that has EVER BEEN DONE . . . and EVERY DANCE that ever WILL be done . . . but you will discover your OWN CREATIVITY.

YOU become the choreographer . . . YOU become the creator . . . and THAT discovery will be far more important than the Dance itself.

For FREESTYLE DISCO, go back to the Chapter on MOVEMENT UNITS and practice ALL of them. FREESTYLE uses every imaginable combination . . . and the object is to interpret the MUSIC. FREESTYLE dancing allows you to DO YOUR THING. Just make sure that YOUR THING is worth doing!

In addition to the LINE DANCE, BODY LANGUAGE and HAND JIVE presented in this chapter, also read the pattern variations of the TWIST under FAD DANCES. Much of the Contemporary BODY LANGUAGE parallels the Step Pattern list from the TWIST.

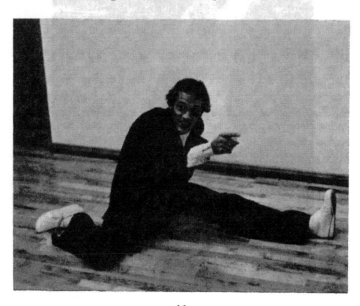

"CALIFORNIA HUSTLE" LINE DANCE (with Variations)

On MAY 14th, 1978, the following LINE DANCE FORMULA was presented at the G.S.D.T.A. WORKSHOP. I announced that with this ONE SHEET OF PAPER, one could teach for SIX MONTHS and never run out of material. Let's explore that statement.

1. A and C are CONSTANT for the LINE DANCE.
   Any B SET, according to level, would complete the LINE DANCE.

2. WITHIN each "B" SET, there is a #2 (2 sets of 8) and a #3 (1 set of 8).
   ANY #2 can be substituted for any other #2. (Same for #3.)

Now, let's forget the LINE DANCE and just select ANY TWO UNITS from any "B" SET (either counts 1 2 3 4 or counts 5 6 7 8). You now have the Basis for a FREESTYLE PATTERN. Repeat your selection. There are TWELVE OBVIOUS COMBINATIONS and by making combinations out of counts 3 4 5 6 you more than double the number.

We can now go ONE STEP FURTHER: Take any of the SYNCOPATIONS and replace your PRIMARY UNITS in another dance pattern that you already know. This could go on for DAYS and you would never run out of material.

LINE DANCES as such will come and go with the times. But there will ALWAYS be room for another version. LINE DANCES are fun and present no PARTNER PROBLEM. They are also useful for learning different foot positions and moves, without worrying about "meshing" with a partner.

(See "GET UP GET DOWN HUSTLE" . . . newest LINE DANCE using these same principles.)

The above information is intended primarily for teachers and advanced students of the UNIVERSAL UNIT SYSTEM. However, with just a minimum amount of study, the information in this text can be invaluable to all.

This LINE DANCE can be done to ANY CONTEMPORARY MUSIC that phrases out to EIGHT sets of EIGHT. (It is also fun danced to SWING MUSIC.)

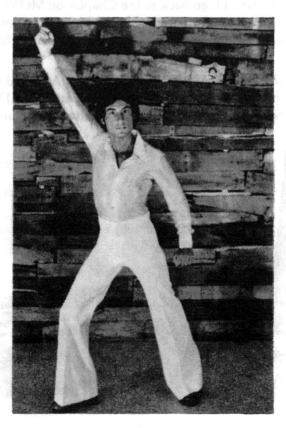

LINE DANCE FORMULA: A + ANY B + C=8 SETS OF 8

FOR G.S.D.T.A. TEACHERS WORKSHOP MAY 14, 1978

A

	1	2	3 & 4	5	6	7 & 8
1st SET #1	B	B	& STEP STEP STEP	F	F	STEP STEP STEP
2nd SET	B	B		F	F	
3rd SET	S	X		S	X	
4th SET	S	X		S	X	
FOOT:	R	L	R L R	L	R	L R L

The TRIPLE could be a SINGLE if desired. SAY: "STEP (touch) instead of STEP STEP STEP

B

	1	2	3	4	5	6	7	8
5th SET #2	S	(B)	S	(B)	S	(B)	(S)	(B)
6th SET	S	(B)	S	(B)	S	(B)	(S)	(B)

(∕) can be in 1st, 5th or whatever.

	1	2	3	4	5	6	7	8
7th SET #3	S	X	X	S	S	hit	S	hit
FOOT:	R	L	R	L	R		L	

"hit" can be knee, "clap," or hip, etc.

B

	1	2	3	4	5 and 6	7	8
5th SET #2	S	S	T	(F)	B T F	S	(B)
6th SET	S	S	T	(F)	B T F	S	(B)

	1	2	3	4	5 and 6	7	8
7th SET #3	S	X	X	S	(F) T (S)	(F) T (S)
FOOT:	R	L	R	L	R	L

43

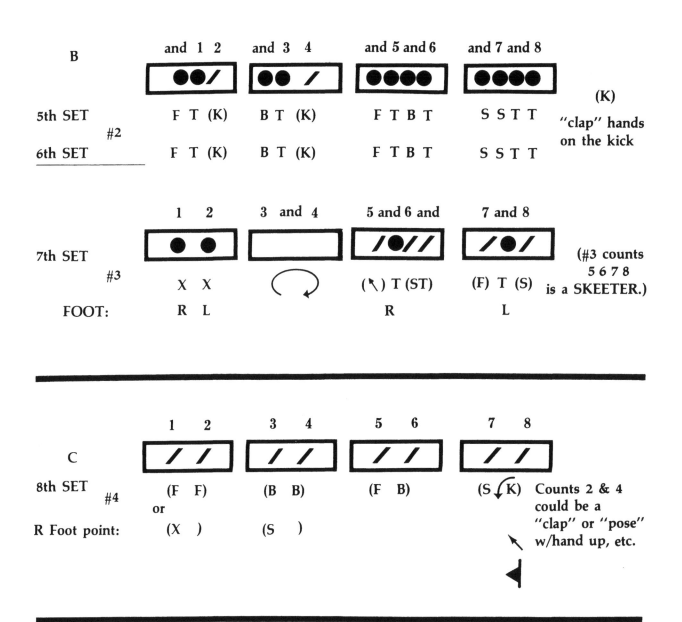

B

| and 1 2 | and 3 4 | and 5 and 6 | and 7 and 8 |

5th SET #2

F T (K)   B T (K)   F T B T   S S T T

(K) "clap" hands on the kick

6th SET

F T (K)   B T (K)   F T B T   S S T T

| 1 2 | 3 and 4 | 5 and 6 and | 7 and 8 |

7th SET #3

X X   (↖) T (ST)   (F) T (S)

FOOT: R L   R   L

(#3 counts 5 6 7 8 is a SKEETER.)

C

| 1 2 | 3 4 | 5 6 | 7 8 |

8th SET #4

(F F)   (B B)   (F B)   (S ↙ K)

or

R Foot point: (X)   (S)

Counts 2 & 4 could be a "clap" or "pose" w/hand up, etc.

44

"GET UP GET DOWN HUSTLE"

By Skippy Blair (Choreographed April, 1978)

- The "GET UP GET DOWN" HUSTLE . . . currently being taught in NITE CLUBS, STUDIOS, SCHOOLS and every place that dancers gather . . . is as versatile as the imagination of the teacher. Long after this particular music is no longer being played, the main body of the routine will serve as a guide for creating NEW routines that fit the day.

- PART 1 . . . is the MAIN THEME of "GET UP GET DOWN" and that part should stay constant. It is choreographed in SETS OF 8.

   Prior to SET #1. There are two sets of 8 to LISTEN . . . and two sets of 8 to get the HIPS going, "LEFT RIGHT, LEFT RIGHT." (Good for learning Body Language and Movement.)

   Set #1. (Maintain the HIP Movement.) Keep LEFT HAND in Neutral (about the waist line). Directions for LEFT HAND and RIGHT HAND are to be done at the same time.

   Set #2. Repeats Set #1 . . . ALL HANDS.

   Set #3. The NEWPORTER . . . SIDE CROSS and SIDE BACK FORWARD & Reverse.

   Set #4. Repeat Set #3.

   Set #5. Both Hands roll to the RIGHT TWICE/ To the LEFT ONCE/ RIGHT HAND UP and repeat through 5 6 & 7 8.

   Set #6. (Only 4 beats.) Roll hands RIGHT TWICE and LEFT TWICE.

   Set #7. BRACE KNEES & stand TALL . . . Point LEFT HAND DOWN to RIGHT SIDE (count 1). Point RIGHT HAND DOWN to LEFT SIDE (count 3 hold 4).

   Stand on one foot and go DOWN DOWN DOWN DOWN for counts 5-6-7-8. (Slap floor on count 8.)

- PART 2 . . . EIGHT SETS OF EIGHT COUNTS that can serve as a guide for teaching ANY DANCE.

   Set #1. Teaches 3 SINGLE RHYTHM UNITS followed by a BLANK to free the other foot.

   Set #2. Repeats Set #1 starting on the other foot.

   Set #3. Teaches TWO DOUBLES and TWO SINGLES. The action between counts 2 & 3 requires DRIVING the C.P.B. to the LEFT. Practice Set #3 by stopping at the end of EVERY UNIT until it is comfortable.

   Set #4. (Same.)

   Set #5. Starts with a SYNCOPATED SINGLE and is a LINK to free the LEFT FOOT. Now do ANY LATIN HUSTLE PATTERN. (Basic only to start.)

   Set #6. One more LATIN HUSTLE PATTERN, plus a BLANK LINK to finish the PHRASE.

   Set #7 and Set #8. Are printed as an exercise to teach NEW YORK HUSTLE. By doing the patterns printed, the student dances both the man's RHYTHM

45

COMBINATION and the lady's RHYTHM COMBINATION. Practice this alone and the COUPLES DANCE will be easy.

The ENTIRE ROUTINE can be danced as a COUPLES DANCE by leaving the MAN'S PART as written and starting the LADY with the LEFT FOOT. To make it fit as a couple, we need only change the LINKS. The FIRST LINK would become a ●● / for the Lady and stay the same for the man. The SECOND LINK, (the BLANK UNIT) we REVERSE the first LINK and have the MAN do the ●● / and the LADY do ● / . . . We are now back to OPPOSITES to complete the NEW YORK HUSTLE.

"GET UP . . . GET DOWN HUSTLE" by SKIPPY BLAIR

Choreographed to "GET UP GET DOWN GET LOOSE"

Album by TEDDY PENDERGRASS

"LIFE IS A SONG WORTH SINGING"

(on 45, flip side of "CLOSE THE DOOR")

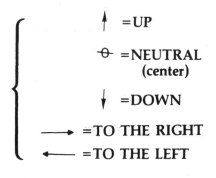

↑ =UP

-θ- =NEUTRAL (center)

↓ =DOWN

⟶ =TO THE RIGHT

⟵ =TO THE LEFT

PART I

	1 2	3 4	5 6	7 8
RIGHT HAND	↑ -θ-	↓ -θ-	→ -θ-	← -θ-
Verbal; 1. & 2.	"UP (snap) (Simultaneous)	DOWN (snap)	OUT (snap)	CROSS" (snap)
LEFT HAND	-θ- -θ-	-θ- -θ-	← -θ-	→ -θ-

NEWPORTER:	1 2	3 & 4	5 6	7 & 8
3.	● ●	●●●	● ●	●●●
	S X	S B F	S X	S B F
FOOT:	R L	R L R	L R	L R L
4.	● ●	●●●	● ●	●●●

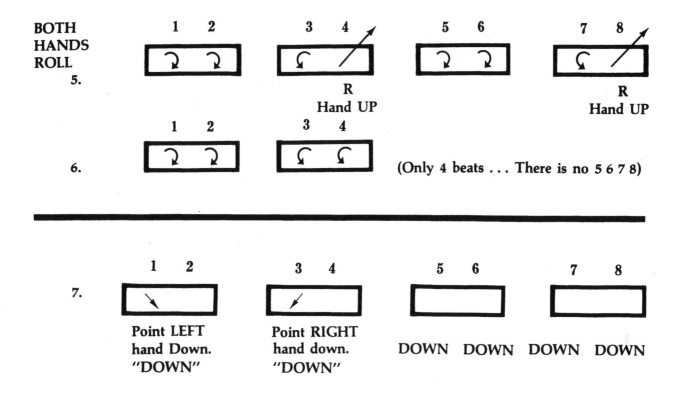

BOTH HANDS ROLL

5.

| 1 | 2 | | 3 | 4 | | 5 | 6 | | 7 | 8 |

R
Hand UP

R
Hand UP

6.

| 1 | 2 | | 3 | 4 |

(Only 4 beats ... There is no 5 6 7 8)

7.

| 1 | 2 | | 3 | 4 | | 5 | 6 | | 7 | 8 |

Point LEFT hand Down. "DOWN"   Point RIGHT hand down. "DOWN"   DOWN   DOWN   DOWN   DOWN

NOTICE that this part of the routine is only 6½ sets of EIGHT counts. You will hear it in the MUSIC and that will help in hearing how to PHRASE OUT Music to fit the dance you want to do. From this last set of eight ... We go into PART 2 of the ROUTINE that conditions the student to do SINGLE RHYTHM and a BLANK ... DOUBLE RHYTHM and SINGLE ... a SYNCOPATED SINGLE "LINK" ... Two LATIN HUSTLE PATTERNS (any direction) ... a BLANK "LINK" to finish the PHRASE ... a DELAYED SINGLE "LINK" to start NEW YORK HUSTLE ... NEW YORK HUSTLE from LADY'S SIDE ... "LINK" MAN'S NEW YORK w/ Syncopated ending.

(See illustrations for PART I — page 49.)

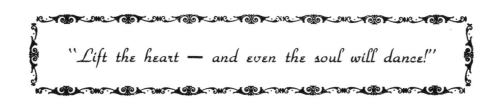

"Lift the heart — and even the soul will dance!"

PART II OF "GET UP GET DOWN HUSTLE"

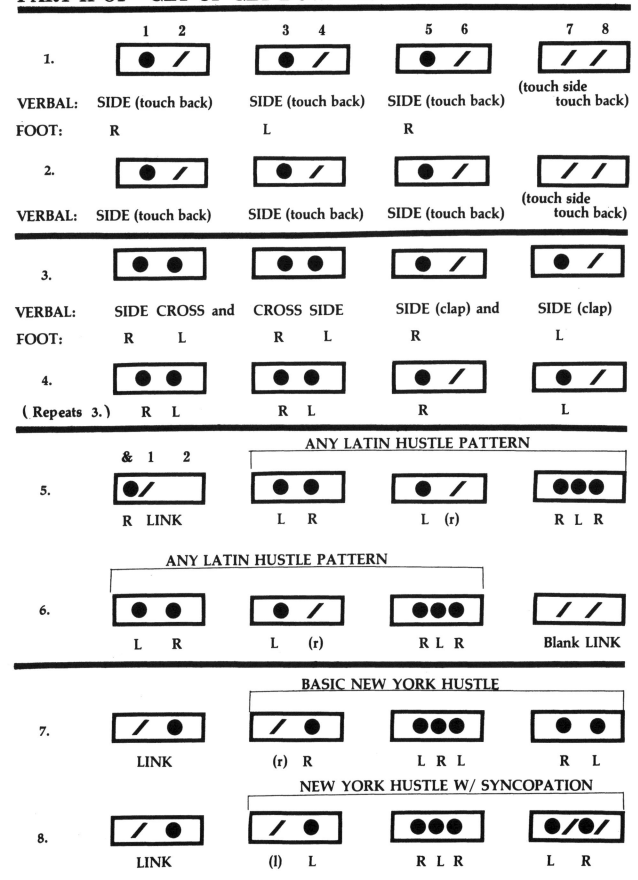

For a BASIC CLASS, I would continue doing LATIN HUSTLE ONLY or work in another dance to fit the phrasing (for SETS 7 and 8). Eliminate the BLANK UNIT at the end of SET 6 and LATIN HUSTLE will phrase to the end.

FOR NIGHT CLUBS or LARGE GROUPS . . . Only do PART 1 & FREESTYLE PART 2.

PART I — Set 1 & 2

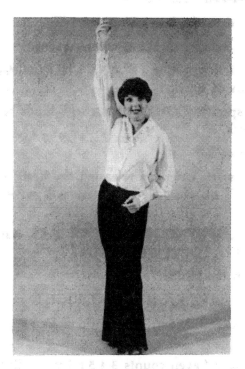 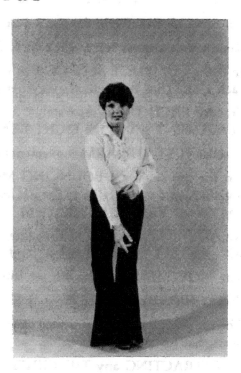

COUNT: **1**   **2**   **3**   **4**

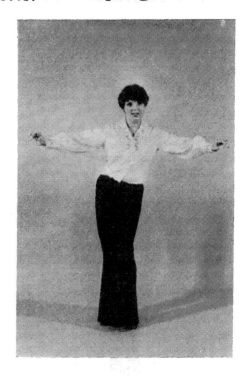 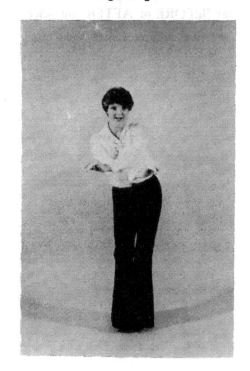

          5   **6**   **7**   **8**

Referring to the BODY LANGUAGE/ DEVELOPING ARMS sheet:

1. The complete 4 sets of 8 counts combines to make an interesting amalgamation.

2. As such, it can be used to replace some of the sets in the GET UP GET DOWN routine.

3. For teaching a CLASS SERIES, pull out TWO UNITS at a time, alternating with SINGLE RHYTHM UNITS to form: "Mini Routines".:

   Do 1st two Units of SET 1 . . . and SINGLE RHYTHM for 5 6 7 8.

   Do SINGLE RHYTHM for 1 2 3 4 of SET 1 and then the last 2 Units of SET 1.

   Repeat that process for EVERY SET. It will make EIGHT different combinations.

4. In doing COMPLETE SETS OF 8, as written . . . Practice putting a BLANK UNIT in between each Unit. That will extend every Set to 16 counts of music.

5. Practice EACH UNIT separately . . . using the specific COUNT that corresponds to the PLACEMENT within the EIGHT BEAT framework.

6. Practice JUST THE ARM movements of each set of 8.

7. On the 3rd set use a BOUNCING MOTION to start. Later try releasing the heels, (feet together) and swing HIPS to the RIGHT to the LEFT on every UNIT. (Heels will move with you doing "Right Left, Right Left.)

   An ADVANCED version of the same set could require SYNCOPATED DOUBLES, starting with the LEFT foot on the first "and" count. (STEP POINT STEP POINT)

8. The MOVEMENT for the 4th set could be just in the HIPS:

   Project HIPS to: LEFT LEFT   RIGHT RIGHT   LEFT RIGHT   LEFT RIGHT.

9. The 1st set of 8 could be repeated starting with the OTHER foot. This would make a set of 16 beats. Set #2 could do the same.

10. By EXTRACTING any TWO UNITS from the page (even counts 3 4 5 6) you will have another whole set of patterns. Extract any two CENTER UNITS and add SINGLE RHYTHM either BEFORE or AFTER the selected two Units.

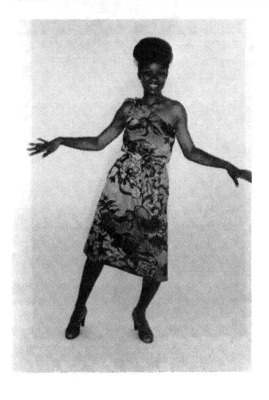
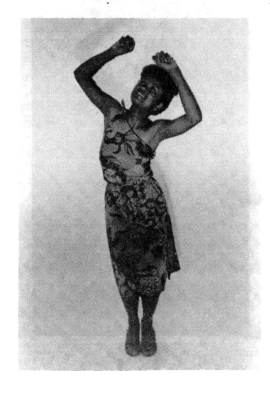

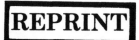

Reprint from Teachers Workshop Conducted for the Bay Area Dance Clinic in Los Altos, Calif., June 10, 1978 by Skippy Blair, UNIVERSAL UNIT SYSTEM.

FREESTYLE AND BODY LANGUAGE

	1	2	3	4	5 and 6	7	8
#1	/	/	/	/	●●●	●	●
	(S)	(T)	(S)	(T)	B T F	T	T
A.	(R)	(R)	(R)	(R)	R L R	L	R
B.	(L)	(L)	(L)	(L)	L R L	R	L

	1 & 2	3	4	5 & 6	7	8
#2	///	/	/	●●●	●	●
	(S)(T)(S)	(F)	(B)	F B T	X	X

ARMS #3 and HANDS

	1	2	3	4	5	6	7	8
	X	OUT	X	OUT	UP	UP	OVER	FRONT
	DOWN		UP		R	L	HEAD	

(FEET TOGETHER, HEELS RELEASED, HEELS MOVING TOGETHER [R   L] .)

#4 HANDS ONLY

	1	2	3	4	5 and 6	7	8
	X	X	X	X	///	/	/

PALMS DOWN

PALMS UP

touch HEELS of hands on (5)   touch FINGER TIPS together on (and) ELBOWS PULL Back on (6)

FISTS TOGETHER (7) POSE R hand up L hand dn (8)

/ =TOUCH, POINT (No Wt. Change)

● =STEP, A WEIGHT CHANGE

Golden State Dance Teachers Association

From Teachers Workshop at Sonora Dance Camp, August, 1978

THE SKEETER

The "SKEETER" . . . A NAME THAT EVOLVED FROM THE OLD "SKEETER RABBIT" made popular by Buddy Schwimmer, 5 year California Rock Champion. This TWO UNIT pattern can be used as an advanced RHYTHM VARIATION in a variety of dances. The SECOND UNIT is the easier of the two & remains the same for all four versions of the pattern. It is a SYNCOPATED SINGLE: "Kick STEP touch"   **/ ● /**

1. Practice JUST the SYNCOPATED SINGLE, alternating LEFT and RIGHT UNITS:

(MOVEMENT is   **UP   DOWN**   )

COUNT:	1 & 2	3 & 4
UNIT:	**/ ● /**	**/ ● /**
VERBAL:	(Kick) STEP (point)	(Kick) STEP (point)
FOOT:	(L) L (R)	(R) R (L) (point can be to the SIDE or forward or back.)

Practice enough to be able to do either a LEFT SYNCOPATED SINGLE . . . or a RIGHT SYNCOPATED SINGLE without thinking about it. It will become as easy as doing a basic SINGLE.

The FIRST UNIT of a SKEETER can be a BLANK UNIT or a different SYNCOPATED SINGLE. A BLANK UNIT is used if you want to START with ONE FOOT FREE and end with the OTHER foot free. You would use the SYNCOPATED SINGLE if you want to start with ONE foot free . . . and end with the SAME FOOT FREE.

(MOVEMENT is   **DOWN DOWN DOWN DOWN**   )

2.   **BLANK UNIT**

COUNT:	1 & 2 &	3 & 4	(Start with either LEFT or RIGHT foot free. OTHER foot will be free at finish.)
UNIT:	**/ / / /**	**/ ● /**	
(FREE Foot):	(F)(T)(S)(T)	(F) T (F)	
VERBAL:	"Kick together Apart together	Kick STEP stamp "	
MOVEMENT:	D D D D	U D	

(Note that there is only ONE STEP in the whole four beats.)

3. SYNCOPATED SINGLE

COUNT:	1 & 2 &		3 & 4	

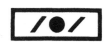

(can also start with LEFT foot free. Will then END with Left foot free.)

FOOT: (R) R (L) (L)   (L) L (R)

VERBAL: "Kick together   Apart together   Kick STEP stamp "

MOVEMENT: D D D D   U   D

(Note that there are TWO steps . . . one in each Unit.)

Any of these combinations would be good in FREESTYLE DISCO.

Also using #2., starting with the LEFT foot free makes an excellent pattern in LATIN HUSTLE. Put the girl in Cradle position. Face forward on count ONE . . . turn ¼ turn RIGHT for count TWO and back to facing forward for counts THREE and FOUR . . . then add the 5 & 6.

D=DOWN
U=UP

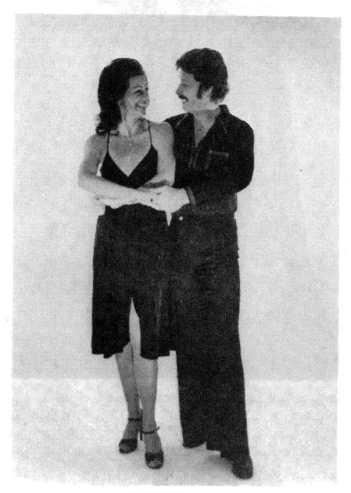

COUNTS: 1 & 3

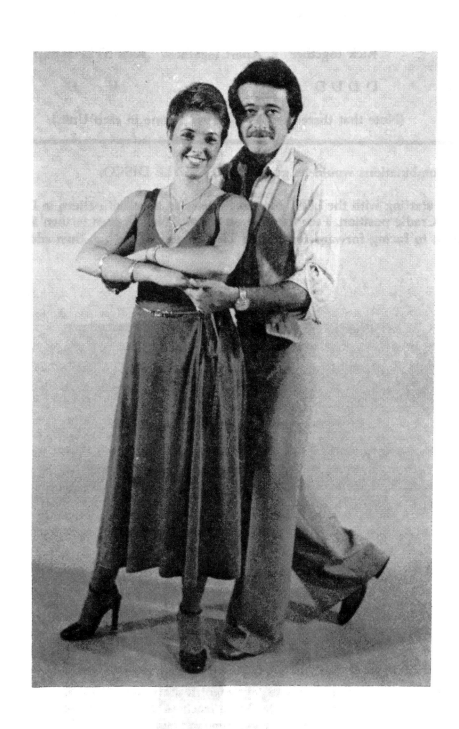

Chapter VII

DISCO . . .
COUPLES DANCING

Standard, traditional dances that have withstood the test of time have one thing in common. They start with a particular RHYTHM PATTERN and then add and expand to include RHYTHM VARIATIONS, SYNCOPATIONS and STYLE VARIATIONS as the patterns become progressively more complicated.

CONTEMPORARY DANCES of the late 70s find a NEW NAME for each RHYTHM COMBINATION. Thus, with just an exchange of RHYTHM UNIT, the SPANISH HUSTLE becomes the LATIN HUSTLE or the LATIN HUSTLE becomes the NEW YORK HUSTLE. The STYLE changes with each area of operation. The RIGHT WAY is always the way its being done wherever YOU go dancing. It would be difficult . . . and pointless . . . to describe each of these dances as a separate dance. ALL three of these dances have been condensed into ONE FORM with varying RHYTHM and STYLE VARIATIONS under the one heading of NEW YORK HUSTLE. The three mentioned rhythm patterns all came out of NEW YORK and so we have classified them all under that one heading . . .

- NEW YORK HUSTLE . . . (the OPPOSITE FOOT HUSTLE). Man starts with his Left foot and the Lady starts with her Right foot, the same as for any of the Standard Social Dances. (See patterns under NEW YORK HUSTLE.)

- LATIN HUSTLE . . . (the SAME FOOT HUSTLE) started on the WEST COAST and had little similarity to its namesake on the East Coast. BOTH partners start with the LEFT FOOT, which makes it unique among couples dances.

The Basic Pattern of BOTH Hustles combines ALL THREE RHYTHM UNITS, unlike the SALSAS which make an entire Dance out of ONE & sometimes TWO RHYTHM UNITS.

Salsa means "Sauce." It is DISCO DANCING with a Latin flavour. During the research for the dance, questioning twenty different teachers and dancers, produced twenty different answers to exactly what SALSA is. More teachers than not responded that SALSA was MUSIC and NOT A DANCE. If we go back in time to when ROCK was first being danced, those same people told us that "ROCK IS NOT A DANCE . . . IT IS MUSIC."*

> * Our ROCK CURRICULUM for GSDTA served teachers nationwide for more than ten years.

Thru the years, we have been in a position that demanded that we know the trends in dancing almost before they happened. Being able to identify that "essence" in a new dance is our stock in trade. Since the reputation of the Association is founded on TEACHER'S TRAINING, professionals look to us for the answers to "WHAT'S NEW? . . . and HOW DO WE TEACH IT?"

Dancing STARTS with the music . . . and the masses dance to that music. They feel certain recurring rhythms and moves that crystallize with repetition into something identifiable.

The SALSA, as music, has been with us for quite some time. The DANCE itself is just coming into its own (1978). With each new era comes an ESSENCE that, once isolated, makes it easy to develop a pattern structure, complete with variations.

The fascinating part of SALSA is that there are four distinctive styles that have emerged. By separating the RHYTHM VARIATIONS, the dancer literally covers the spectrum of the SALSA FEELING. These rhythms can be arranged and rearranged to incorporate all four styles to the SAME TEMPO of music.

- SALSA VALIENTE . . . a series of DOUBLE RHYTHM UNITS that amount to little walking steps, stepping on every beat. A highly stylized version of the basic social dance that has been popular in Mexico for many years. It's STREET NAME is "THE ROPE" so named for the numerous arm loops and underarm turns and wraps. (See patterns . . . this chapter.)

- SALSA PICADO . . . little TRIPLE RHYTHM UNITS with the "Rock" or "break" on the "and" count between the beats. (Resembles Mambo, but a closer look discovers the difference in the MOVEMENT and the timing.)

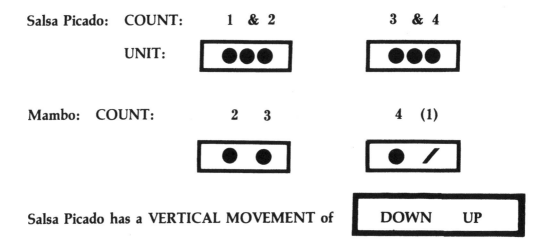

Mambo has HORIZONAL MOVEMENT forward, back or to the side.

- NEWPORTER SALSA . . . alternates DOUBLE and TRIPLE RHYTHM UNITS and is particularly popular in California. STREET NAME is DISCO SWING. (See patterns . . . this chapter.)

- SALSA SUAVE . . . (A Dancers Dance)

Dance aficionados may relate to Salsa Suave as a Rhythm and/or Style variation of Mambolero or International Rumba. The dance "BREAKS" on TWO, the same as Cha Cha or Mambo. It has the feeling of a stepped-up Bolero using DELAYED SINGLES instead of basic SINGLE RHYTHM. It feels and looks very sophisticated and is compatible with Ballroom dancing.

SALSA SUAVE:

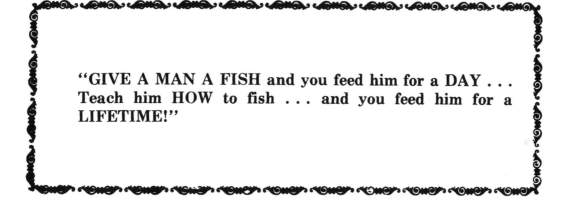

SIDE BASIC:	F	B	(S)	S	B	F	(S)	S
FOOT:	L	R	(L)	L	R	L	(R)	R
HIP MOVES:	R	L	(L)	R	L	R	(L)	L
VERBAL:	"BREAK	STEP	(dig)	STEP	BREAK	STEP	(dig)	STEP"

The CUBAN HIP movement is accented on the "dig step" as the hip moves out with the FREE foot. (All of the Cha Cha patterns will work in Salsa Suave by substituting a DELAYED SINGLE for the TRIPLE RHYTHM UNITS.)

"GIVE A MAN A FISH and you feed him for a DAY . . . Teach him HOW to fish . . . and you feed him for a LIFETIME!"

To paraphrase the above . . .

That's how we feel about the UNIVERSAL UNIT SYSTEM:

"Teach a man a NEW DANCE and he has only learned one new dance. . . . Teach him the UNIT SYSTEM and he will forever be Contemporary in his time."

Contemporary Couples Dances would not be complete without the TWO STEP, TANGO HUSTLE and CONTEMPORARY FOXTROT. These three dances are so intermingled that it is sometimes difficult for an untrained eye to differentiate. The three dances mix well . . . much the same as the Standard dances of Foxtrot and Swing.

- TWO STEP gets its name from the quick little steps that make up the 1st half of the TRIPLE RHYTHM UNIT. The ESSENCE of the Two Step is the ROCK BACK on the count of ONE. The BASIC MOVEMENT is | UP and UP. | TWO STEP is frequently confused with SAMBA.

TWO STEP:

COUNT:	1 & 2			3 & 4		
UNIT:	● ● ●			● ● ●		
DIRECTION:	B F S			B F S		
MOVEMENT CPB:	Up Up			Up Up		

SAMBA:

COUNT:	1 &a 2			3 &a 4		
UNIT:	● ●●			● ●●		
DIRECTION:	S B F			S B F		
MOVEMENT CPB:	Down Down			Down Down		

- CONTEMPORARY FOXTROT . . . alternates DOUBLE and SINGLE RHYTHM with a hint of an | UP DOWN | Movement. Conversation position and Reverses . . . Oversways and Dips . . . all combine to make up the Foxtrot of the Day.

COUNT:	1 2	3 4	5 6	7 8
UNIT:	● ●	● /	● ●	● /

(The fundamental RHYTHM PATTERN for Contemporary Foxtrot is the same as Tango Hustle.)

- TANGO HUSTLE . . . is distinguished by exaggeration of the | UP DOWN |

Movement and the distinctive arm styling reminiscent of the Valentino era. Many of the basic patterns are identical to those of Contemporary Foxtrot. (See patterns . . . this chapter.)

＜=Conversation Position
F=Forward
S=Side
B=Back
( )=No weight

TANGO HUSTLE

Tango Hustle is a FUN dance inspired by the movie SATURDAY NIGHT FEVER. At times it almost seems a spoof on Tango . . . and yet when you really get INTO the dance . . . it is something very special. The UP DOWN of the Basic Movement starts feeling like a ROLLING sensation. This Dance also makes a great SHOW.

COUNT:	1	2		3	(4)	&	5	6		7	(8)

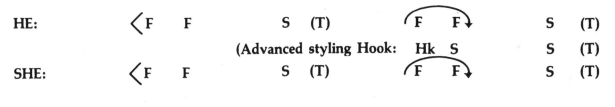

1. BASIC STEP										
HE:	＜F	F	S	(T)	＞	F	F	S	(T)
SHE:	＜F	F	S	(T)	／	F	F	S	(T)
Arms:	"Roll	and	Roll	and	Down	and	Stay	."

(Pattern starts in Conversation Position & reverses direction on count 5.)

2. WALKAROUND (or HOOK TURN)

HE:	＜F	F	S	(T)	⌒F	F↓	S	(T)
			(Advanced styling Hook:	Hk	S		S	(T)
SHE:	＜F	F	S	(T)	⌒F	F↓	S	(T)

TANGO KICK

HE:	＜F	F	F	(K)	&	F	F	B	(T)
SHE:	＜F	F	F	(K)		F	F	B	(T)

(Both RIPPLE forward on the "and" between 5 & 6.)

4. The VALENTINO DRAG

COUNT:	1	2		3	4		5	6		(7)	(8)

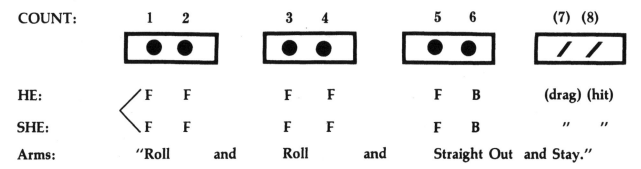

HE:	＜F	F	F	F	F	B	(drag)	(hit)
SHE:	＜F	F	F	F	F	B	"	"
Arms:	"Roll	and	Roll	and	Straight Out	and Stay."

5. TRAVOLTA KICK

COUNT:	1	2		3	&	4		5	6		7	(8)
HE:	F	F		F	B	T		F	F		B	(drag)

(Both partners (Kick) forward with the INSIDE foot on 4.)

SHE:	F	F		F	B	T		F	F		B	(drag)

6. QUICK FAN & DIP

COUNT:	1	2		3	4		5	6		7	8

(from CLOSED POSITION into RIGHT PARALLEL into CLOSED.)

HE:	F	B		B	F		B			F	
VERBAL:	"ROCK"	STEP"		"FAN	AND"		"DIP"			"RETURN"	
							"DIP"			"RETURN"	
SHE:	B	F		F	F		F			B	

7. RHYTHM BREAKS: (all DOUBLE RHYTHM "WALKS" ... "CHASSES" ... ROCKING STEPS ... We add RHYTHM BREAKS to make patterns phrase or to LINK one pattern to another ... or one DANCE to another.

COUNT:	1	2		3	4	
	S	T		S	T	
	F	B		F	B	(Rocking Step or Pivot)

Rhythm Breaks can be done in any dance.

8. FLASH BREAKS include the DEATH DROP ... TORPEDO ... CLIMB ... FREEZE ... and many other Breaks that are compatible with all of the other Contemporary Dances.

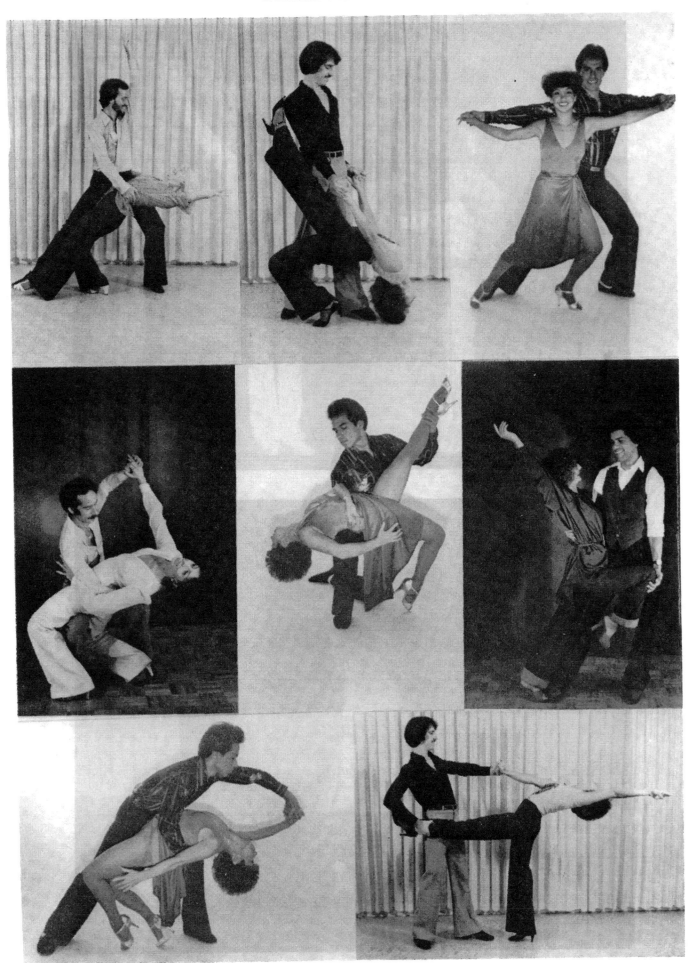

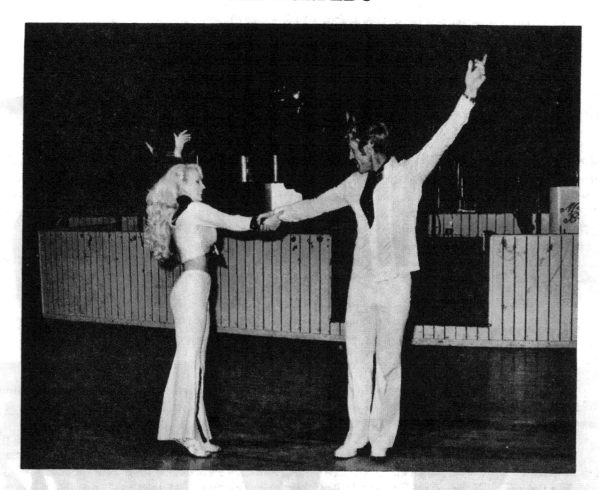

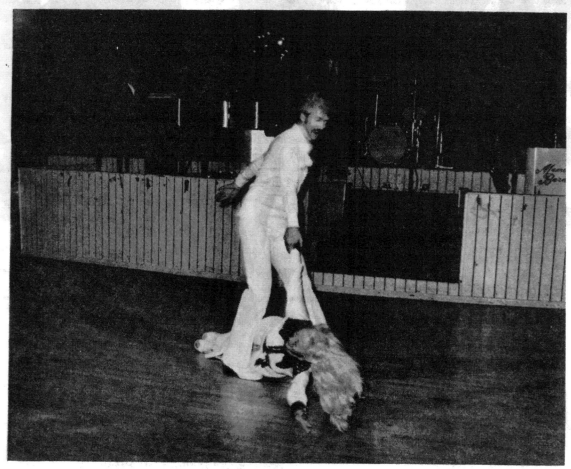

SALSA VALIENTE (THE ROPE)

SALSA VALIENTE is a fun dance. Picture the upright posture of a Matador, picking up his feet with every step. The RHYTHM PATTERN is DOUBLE DOUBLE, a TWO UNIT PATTERN of little marching steps, stepping on every beat. The ARM MOVEMENTS are responsible for dubbing this dance THE ROPE.

SALSA VALIENTE is done with the head held high and a feeling of lifting the head toward the ceiling. FEEL UP!! The MOVEMENT is a little different in that it LOWERS on the first count, and then climbs through count FOUR. It is as if one steps DOWN into a hole and then CLIMBS up and out. At a basic level, it can be done without the climb ... but the EXCITING FEELING of the dance is achieved through this rolling, climbing feeling that extends through BOTH UNITS.

First, practice the RHYTHM PATTERN in place, stepping out the rhythm to the music. Become familiar with the FEELING of the dance by practicing the BASIC MOVEMENT.

Then practice moving FORWARD for four counts ... then BACKWARD for four counts. It will be easy to get the feet moving to the rhythm pattern by just marching to the music. The VERBAL pattern should be the MOVEMENT: DOWN, UP, UP, UP ... This will create a feeling of MOVEMENT in the dance.

Each pattern will start with the man's LEFT foot and the lady's RIGHT foot on count ONE. All patterns listed are danced in two hand position. (Lady dances natural opposite unless otherwise stated.)

SALSA VALIENTE can be danced as a COUPLES DANCE or can be done in formation. If used as a MIXER, the MEN should be facing the CENTER of the circle to start. Ladies will be facing the men. (If there are EXTRA ladies, they may be placed between the couples, to dance their part alone and then move down one partner at the end of each set.)

Those who visit Mexico will recognize the RHYTHM PATTERN as one that has been a basic social dance form in Mexico for many years.

1. BASIC STEP:

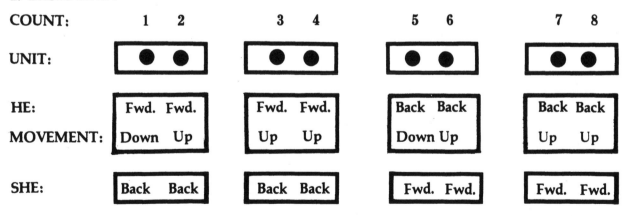

COUNT:	1	2		3	4		5	6		7	8
UNIT:	●	●		●	●		●	●		●	●
HE:	Fwd.	Fwd.		Fwd.	Fwd.		Back	Back		Back	Back
MOVEMENT:	Down	Up		Up	Up		Down	Up		Up	Up
SHE:	Back	Back		Back	Back		Fwd.	Fwd.		Fwd.	Fwd.

(If used as a MIXER, the men should be facing the CENTER of a circle for the first set of EIGHT.)

2. CROSS BODY LEAD: (with Underarm Pivot for the Lady) (Man ¼ turn Left on Count 6).

	1 2	3 4	5 6	and	7 8
HE:	Fwd. Fwd.	Fwd. Fwd.	Back Back	and	Fwd. Fwd.

(Two Hand lead, same as above . . .) (Lead Lady UNDER Left hand on count SIX)

				and	
SHE:	Back Back	Back Back	Fwd. Fwd.	and	Fwd. Fwd.

(Lady pivots LEFT on SIX, reversing position)

3. ONE HAND DRIVE into a CRADLE:

Same as BASIC STEP, above, except man uses ONE HAND (Left hand) following girl's pivot.

	1 2	3 4
MAN'S PATTERN:	● ●	● ●
	Fwd. Fwd.	Fwd. Fwd.

From ONE HAND position: Lady is facing CENTER/ Man STARTS facing Lady, and ENDS facing CENTER.

COUNT:			5	6	7	8
HE:	(Four steps walking around Lady)		Fwd.	Fwd.	Fwd.	Fwd.
SHE:	(Her RIGHT hand loops over head)		Fwd.	Fwd.	Back	Back
					(8 is a CHECK)	

Finish counts 5 6 7 8 by walking AROUND the Lady, CLOCKWISE, stepping Forward, Forward, CHECK★ to finish with BOTH partners facing CENTER. Girl is now in CRADLE POSITION on man's RIGHT SIDE.

4. REVERSE

(In CRADLE POSITION, man reverses action) (Turn girl under arm on count FIVE, releasing Right hand)

COUNT:	1	2	3	4	5	6	7	8
HE:	Back	Back	Back	Back	Back	Fwd.	Fwd.	Fwd.
SHE:	Fwd.	Fwd.	Fwd.	Fwd.	Fwd.	Pivot	Fwd.	Fwd.

(Ready to repeat OR walk 4 steps forward with partner (LOD) and another 4 to new partner.)

There are hundreds of combinations possible in SALSA VALIENTE. All of the patterns in LATIN HUSTLE can be done in DOUBLE RHYTHM. Just walk from one Dance Position to another, keeping time with the music. From OPEN POSITION to CRADLE POSITION . . . from CRADLE to PRETZEL to WHEEL etc. There's no limit.

★This Check is a Forward Step that changes the direction of the CPB to move backward.

LATIN HUSTLE (SAME FOOT HUSTLE)

Probably because of the consistent use of CUBAN HIP MOVEMENT . . . or perhaps because of the Spanish look of the pose in Right Parallel position on the "STAMP" . . . whatever the reason . . . as the numerous Hustles settle down to some kind of firm identification, the SAME FOOT HUSTLE IS the LATIN HUSTLE. (All of the various forms of OPPOSITE foot Hustle have been grouped together under the one heading of New York Hustle (or just plain HUSTLE) (see the "Essence of Contemporary Dance.")

LATIN HUSTLE is a THREE UNIT pattern in its basic form. The BASIC MOVE-MENT is a subtle UP on count ONE and DOWN on count TWO. Practice that movement to the music before starting the patterns. Think of the following rules as individual pieces of information that will make the WHOLE DANCE WORK.

- Movement will be UP DOWN on every Unit.

- BOTH partners start on the LEFT FOOT on count ONE of the pattern.

- The STAMP (gently please) is on count FOUR of the six beat pattern.

- In most instances the STAMP will be in RIGHT PARALLEL position.

- Most of the patterns are danced in a TWO HAND POSITION.

- The LEAD for most of the basic patterns takes place on the FIRST UNIT.

Rather than think in terms of PATTERN . . . practice the POSITIONS of the two partners. This dance moves primarily from ONE POSITION to another on the FIRST UNIT of each pattern. Stand still and move from one position to another without being concerned about the feet. LATER do the same thing using the RHYTHM PATTERN for the LATIN HUSTLE. (These same movements from one position to another can ALL be done in SALSA VALIENTE doing ALL DOUBLE RHYTHM.)

POSITIONS:

1. CRADLE POSITION: SHE is on HIS Right Side . . . BOTH partners facing the same direc-tion. HER arms will be crossed in front of her. His LEFT hand will be in FRONT holding her RIGHT HAND. His RIGHT hand will be in Back of her, holding her LEFT HAND. Get into that position . . . and then practice moving quickly in and out of the position.

2. CRADLE SWITCH: From a CRADLE POSITION move the girl to the man's LEFT SIDE. Do not lift the hand. Keep the arms around the girl. Practice moving her from LEFT to RIGHT until it becomes easy.

3. WHEEL POSITION: Partners are facing opposite walls. To WHEEL to the LEFT, BOTH PARTNERS should have their LEFT ELBOW bent and the RIGHT elbow STRAIGHT. WHEEL to the RIGHT, both partners will have their RIGHT elbow bent and the LEFT elbow STRAIGHT. This puts both partners in a SIDE by SIDE PARALLEL position.

65

4. RIGHT PARALLEL: His RIGHT HIP to HER RIGHT HIP (or Knee to Knee)

5. PRETZEL POSITION: Partners are in Right Parallel. Her LEFT hand is behind her back and her RIGHT hand is extended to the RIGHT. His RIGHT hand holds her LEFT hand. His LEFT hand holds her RIGHT hand.

The man will maneuver the girl into each position on the FIRST UNIT of each pattern. The girl should keep this in mind:

She will turn LEFT under her OWN RIGHT HAND to a CRADLE.

She will turn RIGHT under her OWN RIGHT HAND to a PRETZEL.

If you have been practicing all of these positions, you will be dancing the LATIN HUSTLE in no time at all.

COUNT:	1 2	3 4	5 & 6
UNIT:	● ●	● /	●●●
VERBAL:	"STEP STEP	STEP (Stamp) & STEP THREE TIMES"	
OR	"SWIVEL SWIVEL	STEP (touch) & BACK TOGETHER FORWARD"	
FOOT:	LEFT RIGHT	LEFT (Right)	RIGHT LEFT RIGHT
CUBAN HIP:	RIGHT LEFT	RIGHT (Left)	neutral hip

The Cuban Hip movement is not necessary but is a very good styling.

6. SIDE BY SIDE: Just as the name implies, partners are standing "side by side" the INSIDE hands will be joined. (hand closest to partner.)

7. MACHO POSITION: A PRETZEL with the MAN'S UPPER HAND lifted over his head to rest at the back of his neck.

8. SPANISH POSE: Lady has one hand placed in the small of her back and the other hand placed over her head. The arm is rounded, not straight up. Man's hands hold HER hands as usual, LEFT to RIGHT & RIGHT to LEFT.

9. SHADOW POSITION: Lady in FRONT of the man diagonally to his RIGHT side. (A Shadow CAN be done with the Lady DIRECTLY in front of the man.)

10. BUTTERFLY: (starts with CROSSED HANDS LEFT over RIGHT.)
    If hands are crossed LEFT over RIGHT, the girl will turn LEFT to face the same direction that he faces.
    If the hands are crossed RIGHT over LEFT, she will turn RIGHT to face the same direction that he faces.
    EITHER turn will put the partners in SHADOW POSITION but holding RIGHT HAND to RIGHT HAND and LEFT HAND to LEFT HAND.

The SECOND and THIRD UNITS of each of the following patterns is IDENTICAL. The "STEP (stamp) and STEP THREE TIMES" does not change. Therefore, each pattern will deal only with the FIRST UNIT. Finish each pattern with the same 3 4 5 & 6.

1. BASIC STEP: (Two Hand Lead) say "MARCH MARCH" using CUBAN HIP MOVE-MENT or doing a SWIVEL by stepping to the LEFT on ONE, turn to the right on the ball of the left foot and then step RIGHT on count TWO. Swivel on the ball of the RIGHT foot to face FORWARD for count THREE. Remember that the STAMP will be in RIGHT PARALLEL.

2. CRADLE: HE does a BASIC STEP . . . SHE does a LEFT PIVOT, "FORWARD LEFT and BACK RIGHT" on counts ONE and TWO. Finish with 3 4 5 & 6.

3. CRADLE WALK: From CRADLE POSITION . . . "WALK FORWARD" (Cuban Hip) for ONE and TWO.

   Return to BASIC POSITION from the Cradle Walk on the next "ONE TWO"

Experiment on your own and see how many new variations you can create. Stay with the BASIC RHYTHM PATTERN until you have explored every possible direction that you can turn. THEN experiment with some of the following RHYTHM VARIATIONS:

ANY DOUBLE RHYTHM UNIT can be changed to a DELAYED DOUBLE or a SYNCOPATED DOUBLE. On counts ONE and TWO, instead of "STEP STEP" either partner could do:

COUNT:	1	&	2

UNIT:

VERBAL: "(Kick) STEP STEP"

OR . . .

COUNT:	&	1	&	2

UNIT:

VERBAL: "STEP (Kick) STEP (Kick)"

The SECOND UNIT, the LEFT SINGLE on counts THREE and FOUR, could change from a "STEP (Stamp)" to a "(Kick) STEP (Stamp)", a SYNCOPATED SINGLE.

COUNT:	3	&	4

UNIT:

VERBAL: "(Kick) STEP (Stamp)"

The THIRD UNIT, counts FIVE and SIX could be danced as a SYNCOPATED TRIPLE (similar to a California Shuffle)

COUNT: & 5 & 6 &

UNIT: [●/●/●]

VERBAL: "STEP (Kick) STEP (Kick) STEP"

Numerous other RHYTHM and STYLE VARIATIONS can be achieved in the following manner....

1. FREEZE on count FOUR of a BASIC PATTERN and hold for two extra counts. Finish the pattern with the TRIPLE and you will have a total of EIGHT counts.

2. EXTEND any pattern by adding DOUBLES ... (extra PIVOTS or WALKS) from ANY POSITION. From a PRETZEL POSITION a series of walks will produce a MERRY GO ROUND or a PINWHEEL.

To EXTEND patterns and keep the girl WALKING instead of doing a "Stamp," the man leans away and creates a stronger leverage to keep her moving. He CEASES the leverage the count BEFORE he wants her to "Stamp" and complete the pattern with the TRIPLE.

Practice some of the poses shown here and then create some of your own. Anything goes so long as you maintain the ESSENCE OF THE DANCE.

QUIZ:

1. Both partners start on the _____ foot in Same Foot Hustle.

2. Latin Hustle has how many Units? _____

3. The "Stamp" is on which count of the six beats? _____

4. The lead occurs on which Unit of each pattern? _____

5. We can extend any pattern by adding which kind of Unit? _____

(TEACHERS PLEASE NOTE: The LATIN HUSTLE as shown, continues to be one of the easiest to teach to large groups ... and one of the most successful contemporary dances for mixed ages. Teachers from all areas report an INCREASE in the requests for new material in this particular dance. Grade School Classes, High School, College and even Senior Citizen Classes respond well to the ease of movement and the MARGIN for PERSONAL INTERPRETATION.... We suggest BREAKING to OPEN POSITION on occasion to do some FREE STYLE DISCO and then RETURN to TWO HAND POSITION to continue the LATIN HUSTLE.)

TWO STEP

"TWO STEP" is one of the most popular forms of contemporary social dance. It gets its name from the two little "quick" steps that are observed in the TRIPLE. Many times, dances get tagged with names because of a misconception of what the dance appears to be. Such is the case with TWO STEP. Composed entirely of TRIPLES, it would seem that the dance should be an easy one. It IS easy when understood. Follow these rules & the TWO STEP will be yours.

1. Rock BACK on count ONE of the Triple.

2. Maintain a gentle but noticeable resistance on the "Rock Step." (leverage)

3. Maintain a Basic Movement of UP on count ONE and UP on count TWO. (subtle but definite)

4. Lady dances natural opposite unless otherwise specified.

HE: alternates LEFT TRIPLE — RIGHT TRIPLE
SHE: alternates RIGHT TRIPLE — LEFT TRIPLE

#1. BASIC STEP (Closed Dance Position)

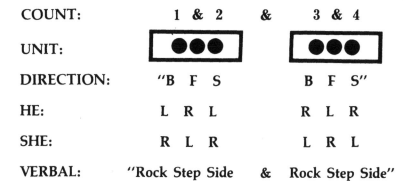

COUNT:	1 & 2	&	3 & 4
UNIT:	●●●		●●●
DIRECTION:	"B F S		B F S"
HE:	L R L		R L R
SHE:	R L R		L R L
VERBAL:	"Rock Step Side	&	Rock Step Side"

#2. TURNING THE BASIC (Left and Right)

a. To Turn LEFT man turns his CPB ¼ turn Left on the 1st unit of a Basic Step (count 2)
b. To Turn RIGHT man turns his CPB ¼ turn Right on the 2nd unit of a Basic Step (count 4)
   (Lady makes ½ a turn LEFT between the Units to walk Forward for counts 2 & 3.)

#3. CROSSING BASIC (closed Dance Position)

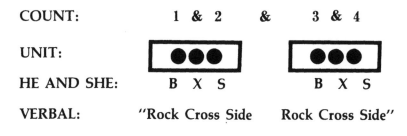

COUNT:	1 & 2	&	3 & 4
UNIT:	●●●		●●●
HE AND SHE:	B X S		B X S
VERBAL:	"Rock Cross Side		Rock Cross Side"

#4. CONVERSATION BASIC

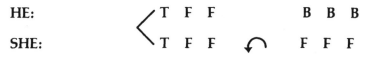

HE:	T F F		B B B
SHE:	T F F		F F F
VERBAL:	"Both Walk Forward & He Walks Back"		

(Lady makes ½ a turn LEFT between the Units to walk Forward for counts 2 & 3.

#5. RIGHT HOOK TURN (clockwise turn)

Pattern starts in conversation position.

COUNT:	1 & 2	&	3 & 4
UNIT:	●●●		●●●
HE:	T F F		HK S F
SHE:	T F F		F F F

HE Hooks the Right foot behind the Left on count 3 and turns CW as she runs around him, also CW.

#6. RUNNING LEFT TURN

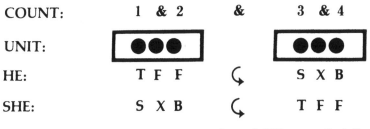

COUNT:	1 & 2	&	3 & 4
UNIT:	●●●		●●●
HE:	T F F	↺	S X B
SHE:	S X B	↺	T F F
VERBAL:	"SHE turns Left and HE turns Left"		

• The C.P.B. moves "FFF" on the "TFF" TRIPLE.
• Repeat pattern several times moving around the room.

#7. UNDERARM TURN (Two Hand Lead)

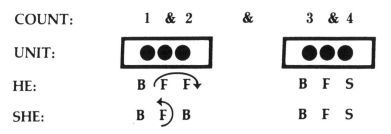

COUNT:	1 & 2	&	3 & 4
UNIT:	●●●		●●●
HE:	B F F↴		B F S
SHE:	B F) B		B F S
VERBAL:	"SHE goes under & Rock Step Side"		

• She goes under her own Right Hand on "&2" as she turns LEFT. There is an exchange of places.

#8. HIS UNDERARM TURN

HE:	B F S	&	B F) B
SHE:	B F S	&	B F F↴
VERBAL:	"Rock Step Side & He goes under"		

• He goes under his OWN RIGHT hand on "and 4"

X = Cross in Front
< = Conversation Position—Partners hinged at inside hip.
T = Together

F = Forward
B = Back
S = Side
CW = Clockwise

70

#9. DOUBLE UNDERARM TURN

HE:	B ⌒F F↓	&	B F) B	
SHE:	B F) B	&	B ⌒F F↓	
VERBAL:	"SHE goes under & HE goes under."			

• In all of the Underarm Turns the hand that is NOT in use is released on the UP BEAT just long enough to complete the turn. Resume two hand position or CLOSE the position by leading the Lady's underarm turn and "catch" her on count 2. Remain in closed position thru count 4.

#10. FALLAWAY CHECK

COUNT:	1 & 2	&	3 & 4
UNIT:	●●●		●●●
HE:	B T F		B T F
SHE:	B T F		B T F

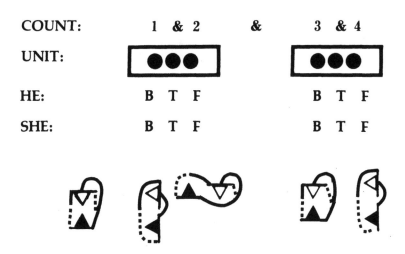

•Starting in Closed Position . . . Both partners swivel to step BACK in Conversation Position on count ONE. Bring the feet together on the "and" count. Swivel to face each other to CHECK FORWARD on count TWO.

•Follow a Fallaway Check with a series of PIVOTS either clockwise or counter-clockwise.

• In leading TWO STEP it is important for the man to maintain a firm but flexible RIGHT HAND. In all of the closed position patterns, his Right Hand will be on his partners back, just below the shoulder blade. Think of it as an extension of your OWN center point of balance.

QUIZ:

1. Contemporary TWO STEP is composed of how many Units?_____

2. He alternates a _____ TRIPLE and a _____ TRIPLE.

3. The BACK ROCK takes place on which count of the TRIPLE? _____

4. A HOOK TURN on a man's RIGHT TRIPLE will turn clockwise or counterclock-wise? _____

5. The Basic Movement of TWO STEP is _____ & _____

NEWPORTER SALSA (DISCO SWING)

The NEWPORTER SALSA was "BORN" in Southern California. It is a combination of closed dancing, similar to a jazzy FOXTROT, which then changes into UNDERARM MOVES which resemble SWING.

It is a real FUN DANCE and quite popular among the vast majority of STREET DANCERS. Isolating the SALSA TRIPLE placed this dance in the SALSA CATEGORY. The NEWPORTER,★ in NEWPORT BEACH was the first CLUB to introduce this new Dance in its PRESENT FORM. Therefore, we christened it: NEWPORTER SALSA . . . BOTH partners walk forward on the DOUBLE RHYTHM steps. Also, the man and woman ALTERNATE the starting walking foot. He walks forward LEFT RIGHT and STEP ROCK STEP . . . then walks forward RIGHT LEFT and STEP ROCK STEP. She does the natural opposite. Without observing the ESSENCE it would be easy to see the CHARACTERISTICS of the dance and think it is SWING.

Doing the NEWPORTER is easy because it PHRASES naturally. It is a FOUR UNIT PATTERN . . . (EIGHT beats of Music.)

Start in CONVERSATION POSITION, hinged at Man's RIGHT hip and Lady's LEFT hip, with both partners ready to walk FORWARD.

1. BASIC STEP and WALKAROUND:

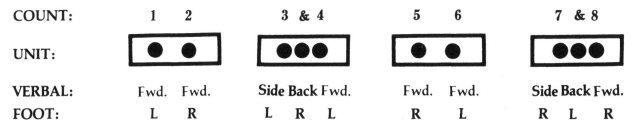

COUNT:	1	2		3 & 4			5	6		7 & 8	
UNIT:	●	●		●●●			●	●		●●●	
VERBAL:	Fwd.	Fwd.		Side	Back	Fwd.	Fwd.	Fwd.		Side	Back Fwd.
FOOT:	L	R		L	R	L	R	L		R	L R

(Lady will be dancing the NATURAL OPPOSITE. On counts FIVE and SIX, partners will be walking around each other in RIGHT PARALLEL POSITION.) Repeat the Pattern.

2. INSIDE ROLL for LADY: (First half of the pattern is identical to #1.)

Second half of pattern LADY TURNS LEFT on count FIVE & SIX as man leads an inside roll. This puts them in ONE HAND . . . OPEN POSITION. The 7 & 8 is completed back in TWO HAND POSITION.

This is the TRANSITION from CLOSED POSITION PATTERNS to OPEN POSITION.

There are endless varieties of directions to go. On Pattern #1 the MAN can do a HOOK TURN on counts 5 & 6 instead of the WALKAROUND. (Pattern would be similar to a RHYTHM VARIATION of TANGO HUSTLE . . . except that the ESSENCE is different. The BASIC MOVEMENT is also different:

TANGO HUSTLE . . . Basic Movement is | UP   DOWN |

NEWPORTER . . . Basic Movement is | DOWN   UP |

★Bob and Sharon Boies of Mr. Roberts Dance Studio in Newport Beach were the Teachers who pioneered the NEWPORTER, (UNIT CARDS and all!!)

To get ready for doing UNDERARM TURNS, the following exercises are suggested. (Particularly helpful for teaching classes.) EVERYONE faces the same wall:

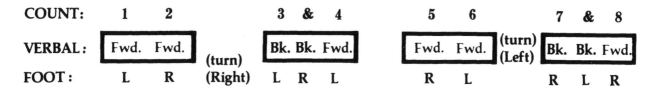

COUNT:	1	2		3	&	4		5	6		7	&	8
VERBAL:	Fwd.	Fwd.	(turn)	Bk.	Bk.	Fwd.		Fwd.	Fwd.	(turn) (Left)	Bk.	Bk.	Fwd.
FOOT:	L	R	(Right)	L	R	L		R	L		R	L	R

This exercise emphasizes that we TURN in the direction of the forward foot. Notice that the first WALK WALK (both forward) STARTS with the LEFT FOOT. The second WALK WALK (both forward) starts with the RIGHT FOOT.

After practicing the above until it becomes easy, it is time to put the pattern together as a couple. Start with a TWO HAND POSITION:

3. UNDERARM TURNS

Man's LEFT FOOT is free. Lady's RIGHT FOOT is free. SHE will go under her own RIGHT hand . . . on count TWO. HE goes under his own RIGHT hand on count SIX.

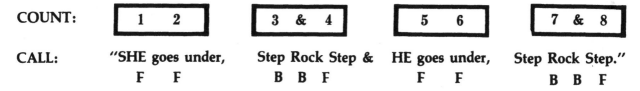

COUNT:	1	2		3	&	4		5	6		7	&	8
CALL:	"SHE goes	under,		Step	Rock	Step &		HE goes	under,		Step	Rock	Step."
	F	F		B	B	F		F	F		B	B	F

Practice Pattern #3, starting from a TWO HAND POSITION until it becomes easy. Then put them together . . . #1 . . . #2 and #3.

4. PIVOTS, GRAPEVINES and other RHYTHM BREAKS work well with the Newporter.

Rules regarding the TRIPLES, help in the creation of new material as well as in executing the patterns presented.

For Newporter Salsa:

- Triples danced in closed position start to the side:

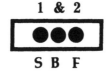

- Triples danced in 2 hand or open position start on a backward step:

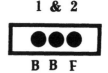

- In BOTH cases the "rock" is on the "and" count.

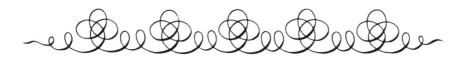

73

NEW YORK HUSTLE
(1978 Vintage)

NEW YORK HUSTLE ... OPPOSITE FOOT HUSTLE, STANDARD BALLROOM HOLD

Man starts with LEFT FOOT ... Lady starts with RIGHT FOOT.

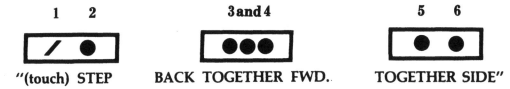

1 2	3 and 4	5 6
"(touch) STEP	BACK TOGETHER FWD.	TOGETHER SIDE"

The ESSENCE of NEW YORK HUSTLE is the DRAMATIC ELEGANCE that seems to literally transport the dancers up and out of themselves. The subtle LIFT on the first beat of every UNIT (counts 1, 3, and 5) gives one the feeling of being "air-borne."

NEW YORK HUSTLE is the most technical of the Contemporary Couples Dances. When it is done properly it is beautiful. When it is danced poorly, it resembles a distorted SWING. Pay attention to the MOVEMENT of the BASICS and you will be well rewarded. The FEELING that comes over a dancer when all of the ingredients get together is overwhelming, and the feeling of NEW YORK HUSTLE is a musical HIGH! (Don't settle for less.)

PRACTICE the DELAYED SINGLES by themselves, counting "ONE two and THREE four."

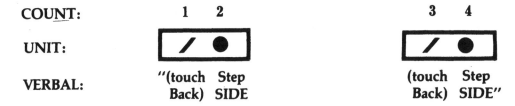

COUNT:

UNIT:

VERBAL:

"(touch   Step
Back)   SIDE

(touch   Step
Back)   SIDE"

(The FREE FOOT should swing like a pendulum, from the C.P.B. If the body is stretched and lifted, the KNEE of the free leg will not have to be bent. Practice that FREE SWING, feeling that the TOP of the pendulum is in the SOLAR PLEXUS (C.P.B.).

Start:

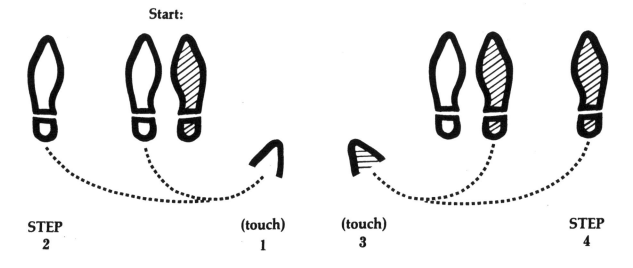

STEP
2

(touch)
1

(touch)
3

STEP
4

NEXT ... PRACTICE THE TRIPLES, alternating "LEFT RIGHT LEFT and RIGHT LEFT RIGHT."

COUNT:	1 & 2	3 & 4
UNIT:	●●●	●●●
VERBAL:	"BACK TOGETHER FORWARD	& BACK TOGETHER FORWARD"
FOOT POS:	4th 1st 4th	4th 1st 4th

The fascinating part of this exercise is to first practice it as stated ... stepping STRAIGHT BACK, then TOGETHER, then FORWARD, until you can alternate the TRIPLES with ease.

NOW, do those SAME TRIPLES on a DIAGONAL. (See floor pattern below.) It LOOKS as if it were a "CROSS BEHIND." It is not. There are TWO MOTIONS that come into play, creating that elegant movement.:

1. The BODY (C.P.B.) is moving BACK and FORWARD, while the SWING of the leg is the SIDE PENDULUM MOVEMENT of the FIRST EXERCISE.

2. The LEG is still swinging from SIDE TO SIDE in a PENDULUM MOVEMENT, as per the FIRST EXERCISE.

3. The C.P.B. stays facing forward toward front wall (or toward partner, if in Dance Pos.).

4. When the TWO MOVEMENTS get together ... it's GREAT!!

Start:

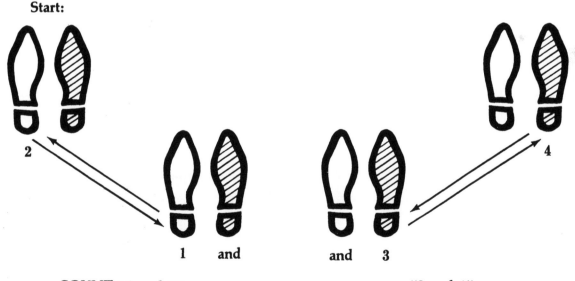

COUNT:"1 and 2"   "3 and 4"

If you will practice the DELAYED SINGLES ... and then the DIAGONAL TRIPLES separately and apart from each other, the SIMILARITY of the movement and the timing should become apparent. This understanding of these two RHYTHM UNITS in the style of NEW YORK HUSTLE makes it easy to see how to SUBSTITUTE one Rhythm for another. These two Rhythms are INTERCHANGEABLE in many variations of patterns.

For Beginners it is suggested that the two TRIPLES be used instead of the DELAYED SINGLE. (Later, alternate them.)

Now we are ready for the THIRD UNIT. It should be practiced alone also.

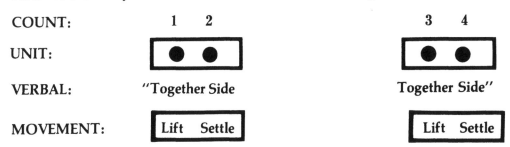

COUNT: 1   2   3   4

UNIT:

VERBAL: "Together Side   Together Side"

MOVEMENT: Lift Settle   Lift Settle

(Please note that the movement on 2 and 4 is NOT DOWN. It is just LESS lifted than the movement on 1 and 3. Think NEUTRAL on 2 and 4.)

Practice the above movement and pattern, starting first with the LEFT FOOT and traveling to the RIGHT. Then stop and start again, starting with the RIGHT FOOT and traveling to the LEFT.

If ALL THREE UNITS have been practiced ALONE, it will then be easy to put the pieces together to form the Dance:

1. BASIC STEP in NEW YORK HUSTLE . . . a THREE UNIT PATTERN:

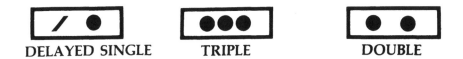

DELAYED SINGLE   TRIPLE   DOUBLE

Both partners facing each other in CLOSED DANCE POSITION. His RIGHT HAND is an extension of his OWN C.P.B. By moving his OWN C.P.B. as he dances, his LEAD will be transmitted to his partner WITHOUT excess pushing and pulling. Remember that a LEAD is an INDICATION of direction.

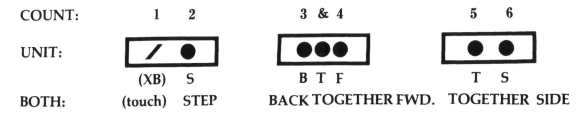

COUNT: 1   2   3 & 4   5   6

UNIT:

           (XB) S   B T F   T S

BOTH: (touch) STEP   BACK TOGETHER FWD. TOGETHER SIDE

2. OPEN BASIC . . . Pattern is the same as #1. with the exception that the 2nd UNIT, (the BACK TOGETHER FORWARD) is facing the man's RIGHT WALL.

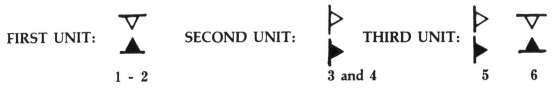

FIRST UNIT: SECOND UNIT: THIRD UNIT:

          1 - 2   3 and 4   5   6

The ARM LEAD to go from the 1st UNIT to the 2nd UNIT is a CIRCULAR MOVEMENT, CLOCKWISE on count THREE and COUNTERCLOCKWISE on count FOUR. This puts both partners in a SIDE BY SIDE position for the "BACK TOGETHER FORWARD."

The last UNIT is a "FORWARD SIDE" for both partners. To add style to the Lady's pattern, she should pull her LEFT SHOULDER BACK on count FIVE as she steps FORWARD. This action will snap her to face her partner as she steps SIDE on count SIX. (Practice this movement over and over again.)

3. WORKING BASIC . . . (and GIRLS . . . guess who's doing the WORK? . . . We are!)

    1. Man does a BASIC PATTERN (as shown in #1.)

    2. Lady does an OPEN BASIC (pattern #2.)

    3. The LEAD is a PUSH & PULL on counts THREE & FOUR.

    4. The SHOULDER styling for the Lady gets more pronounced in this one. (Emphasize movement from pattern #2.)

Positions of Partners on Specific Units:

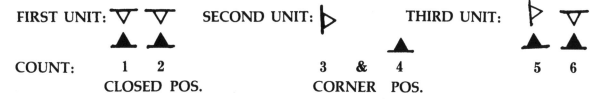

FIRST UNIT: SECOND UNIT: THIRD UNIT:

COUNT: 1   2   3 & 4   5   6

    CLOSED POS.   CORNER POS.

4. An EXTENDED WORKING BASIC (with Underarm PIVOT for LADY).

We can EXTEND any Pattern by adding an extra DOUBLE RHYTHM UNIT . . . or just by REPEATING a DOUBLE RHYTHM UNIT that is already in the Pattern. To extend this SIX BEAT PATTERN, we make it into an EIGHT BEAT PATTERN (from a THREE UNIT to a FOUR UNIT PATTERN). This is particularly helpful in choreographing to specific music. By adding extra UNITS we can make a particular pattern PHRASE to the music.

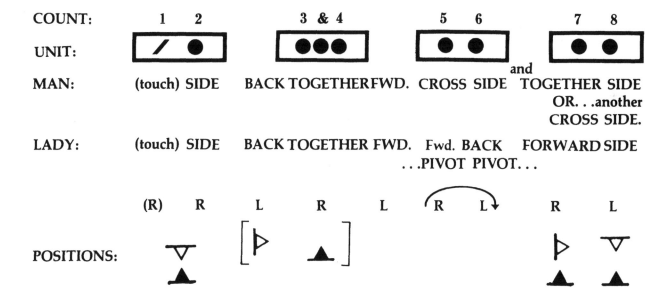

COUNT:	1	2	3 & 4	5	6	7	8

5. LEFT and RIGHT TURNS (BASIC).

• LEFT TURNS ... Doing a BASIC PATTERN (#1) the man makes a gradual turn LEFT on COUNT FIVE (¼ turn Left).

It is important to practice BASIC PATTERNS without turning, in order to cement the TECHNIQUE that makes the patterns work. After that, floor craft is learned by being able to maneuver around the floor, either turning LEFT or RIGHT in your basic patterns.

• RIGHT TURNS are achieved by turning RIGHT on count FOUR of the SIX beat pattern ... or on count SIX of an EIGHT BEAT PATTERN.

6. CROSS BODY LEAD

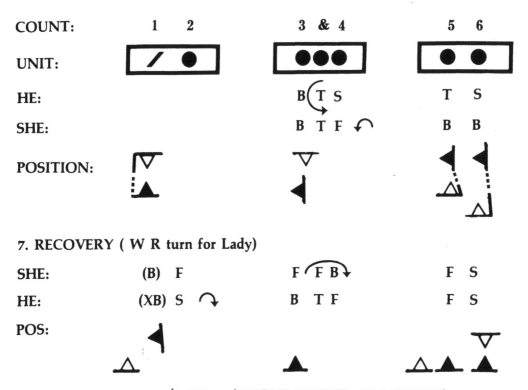

7. RECOVERY (W R turn for Lady)

(LEFT and RIGHT UNDERARM TURNS)

LADY'S TURNS

1. From a Corner Position, Lady turns LEFT (CCW)* on count THREE.

She makes a RIGHT TURN on count TWO or in an ADVANCED FORM, the man leads her into a RIGHT TURN on the "AND" count after the THREE. This is particularly effective when the man's LEAD is a STRAIGHT DOWN SWING of the arm into a CLOCKWISE FULL CIRCLE starting on THREE.

MAN'S TURNS

2. MAN turns LEFT under his own arm (also from a RECOVERY), on count TWO.

This is not an easy turn but can be accomplished with practice. For MAN'S UN-DERARM TURNS, the KEY is to release the TENSION or RESISTANCE as he goes under. This releases, rather than tightens, the tension between the two partners ... so that he can complete his turn without interference.

MAN'S RIGHT TURN can be accomplished on count FOUR or on count THREE. The THREE becomes a HOOK TURN and is an ADVANCED MOVE. Practicing EACH UNIT separately and apart from the whole pattern ... makes ADVANCED MATERIAL easy.

*CCW=counter clockwise

78

POSITION CHART

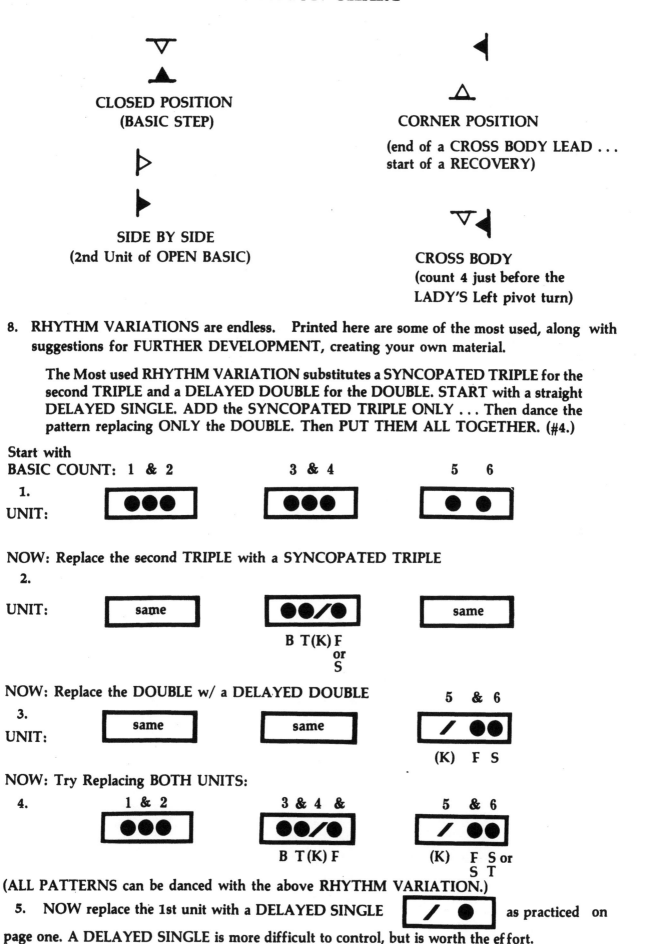

CLOSED POSITION
(BASIC STEP)

CORNER POSITION

(end of a CROSS BODY LEAD . . .
start of a RECOVERY)

SIDE BY SIDE
(2nd Unit of OPEN BASIC)

CROSS BODY
(count 4 just before the
LADY'S Left pivot turn)

8. RHYTHM VARIATIONS are endless. Printed here are some of the most used, along with suggestions for FURTHER DEVELOPMENT, creating your own material.

The Most used RHYTHM VARIATION substitutes a SYNCOPATED TRIPLE for the second TRIPLE and a DELAYED DOUBLE for the DOUBLE. START with a straight DELAYED SINGLE. ADD the SYNCOPATED TRIPLE ONLY . . . Then dance the pattern replacing ONLY the DOUBLE. Then PUT THEM ALL TOGETHER. (#4.)

Start with
BASIC COUNT: 1 & 2   3 & 4   5   6

1.
UNIT:

NOW: Replace the second TRIPLE with a SYNCOPATED TRIPLE

2.
UNIT: same   ●●/●   same
                               B T(K) F
                                  or
                                  S

NOW: Replace the DOUBLE w/ a DELAYED DOUBLE   5   &   6
3.
UNIT: same   same   / ●●
                                               (K) F S

NOW: Try Replacing BOTH UNITS:
4.   1 & 2   3 & 4 &   5   &   6
               ●●●   ●●/●   / ●●
                               B T(K) F   (K)   F S or
                                                     S T

(ALL PATTERNS can be danced with the above RHYTHM VARIATION.)

5.   NOW replace the 1st unit with a DELAYED SINGLE   / ●   as practiced on

page one. A DELAYED SINGLE is more difficult to control, but is worth the effort.

Some More ADVANCED RHYTHM COMBINATIONS . . .

6. Try replacing the TRIPLE with a SYNCOPATED TRIPLE:

COUNT: & 3 & 4 &

UNIT: ● ／ ● ／ ●

VERBAL: STEP(point)STEP(point)STEP

(CALIFORNIA SHUFFLE from any position.)

7. From a CORNER POSITION, the LADY can do a RIPPLE by substituting a SINGLE RHYTHM UNIT for counts 3 & 4.

COUNT: 3   4   5   6

UNIT: ● ／   &   ● ●
VERBAL: STEP (KICK)   (RIPPLE)   F   S

8. Another popular RHYTHM VARIATION is to replace the DOUBLE with a SYNCOPATED DOUBLE:

COUNT: & 5 & 6

UNIT: ●／●／

VERBAL: STEP(point)STEP(point)

ALL OF THE RHYTHM VARIATIONS can be done in any BASIC or ADVANCED PATTERN. It is easiest to practice RHYTHM VARIATIONS in BASIC PATTERNS ... and COMPLICATED PATTERNS using BASIC RHYTHMS. Eventually, the two are interchangeable.

9. A GRAPEVINE is a series of twisting moves that alternate stepping Back/Side/Forward/Side, traveling either Left or Right.
   The GRAPEVINE can be done in a TRIPLE as well as in the following version, which is a substitute for the DOUBLE RHYTHM UNIT (replace with EXTENDED DOUBLE).

COUNT: 5 & 6 &

UNIT: ● ● ● ●   (Four Steps to Two Beats of Music.)

VERBAL: CROSS, SIDE,CROSS Bk, SIDE,
            X   S   XB   S
LADY: CROSS Bk, SIDE, CROSS,   SIDE
          XB   S   X   S

10. The Rhythm of the STREET HUSTLE is also used as a variation of NEW YORK HUSTLE (see Street Hustle).

COUNT: & a 1   2   3 & a 4   5   6

UNIT   ●● ●   ● ●●   ● ●

QUIZ: 1. How many Units in New York Hustle ?_____

        2. We can use a variety of Rhythms on the second unit. Show at least two.
        _____   _____

        3. There is a subtle movement on Count one of every Unit. It is _____

        4. In the pendulum action, the top of the pendulum is located at the _____

80

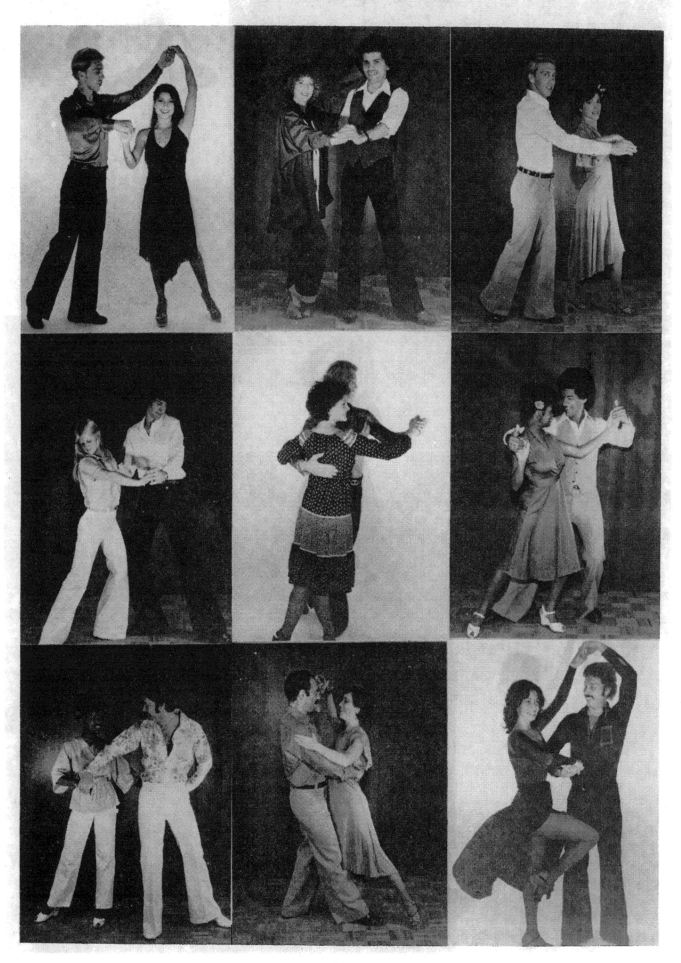

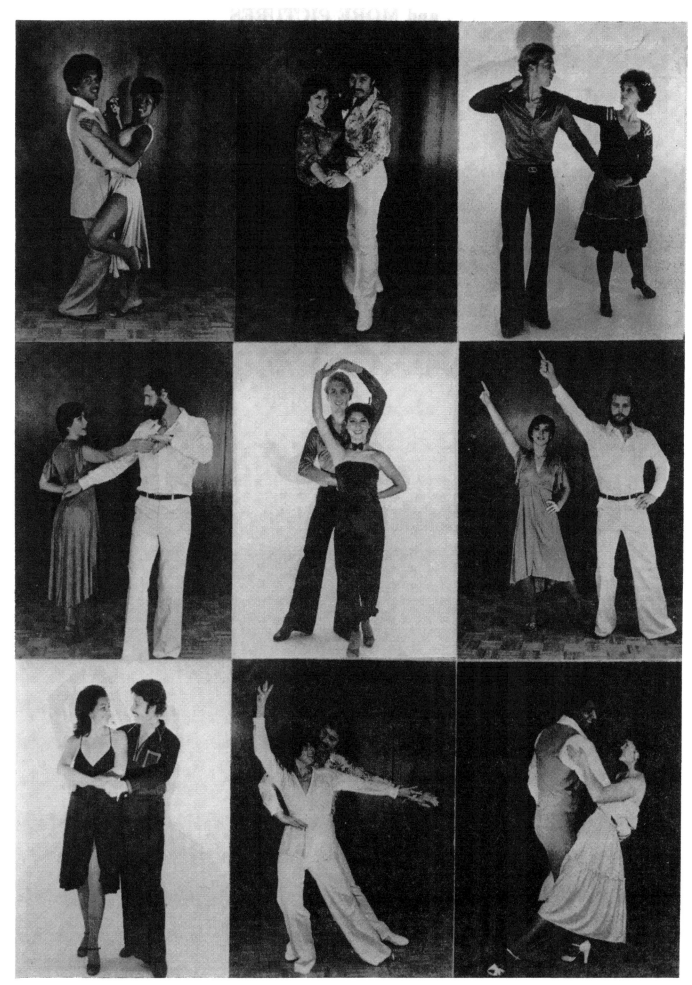

Chapter VIII

THE STANDARD BALLROOM DANCES

The Standard Ballroom Dances are those dances which have not only survived the test of time but have been danced continuously since their inception.

FOXTROT, WALTZ, TANGO, SAMBA, RUMBA, CHA CHA and SWING are considered to be the seven standards.

Each of these dances contributes some MOVEMENT . . . RHYTHM CHANGE . . . BODY STYLING . . . or CONTROL that gives a dancer TOTAL FORM. A dancer who understands the similarities as well as the differences of all of the social standard dances can readily recognize and adapt as new dances arrive on the scene.

Contemporary Social Dance refers not only to the new dances of the day . . . but to the current styling of the standard basic dances.

Frequently, people are not aware of the GRADUAL, but CONTINUOUS CHANGE that takes place in all of the standard dances.

The dance breakdowns presented in this chapter will give you a foundation for the basics . . . along with the key information that will lead you to innumerable pattern variations.

The understanding of all of the dances becomes elementary if the student understands the BASIC UNIT STRUCTURE of the dance. Re-read Chapters I and II until the language of the dance is second nature. Studying the TERMINOLOGY in Chapter XV will also add greatly to your dancing knowledge.

Don't be content with just reading a specific dance. Find out all there is to know about dancing itself. The rewards in the feeling of self accomplishment and the feeling of self expression are beyond description.

FOXTROT

In New York in the early 1900's (1914-1916) a musical comedy star by the name of Harry Fox did a series of fast walking steps to music, that developed into what we know as FOXTROT.

Basic FOXTROT in any era, refers to the current medium tempo, closed position dancing, danced to 4/4 time music. The STYLE changes according to the type of music, the age of the dancers, and the location of the dance: (Nite Club . . . Ballroom . . . Discotec . . . Country Club . . . Private party etc.) Whatever the style, one similarity binds them all together. They are all composed of two PRIMARY RHYTHM UNITS . . . SINGLE and DOUBLE RHYTHM. Following the methods of the Universal Unit System, all of the variations of Foxtrot become very easy to understand.

BEFORE DOING THE PATTERNS, read Chapter I and II. KNOW THE FOOT POSITIONS AND THE UNITS and all else will be mere arrangement.

The UNITS used in the following FOXTROT PATTERNS are:

SINGLE RHYTHM :   STEP on count one and TOUCH (brush) on count two
                    ONE WEIGHT CHANGE to two beats of music

DOUBLE RHYTHM :   STEP on count one and again on count two . . .
                    TWO WEIGHT CHANGES to two beats of music

THE FOOT POSITIONS THAT WE ARE GOING TO USE ARE:

FIRST: Feet together   SECOND: feet directly apart and
     FOURTH: A STRAIGHT WALKING STEP either forward or back.

Armed with these TWO UNITS and THREE FOOT POSITIONS, we can do an infinite variety of steps in FOXTROT:

Before doing ANY PATTERNS . . . Practice the individual RHYTHM UNITS in place . . . and moving in different directions. When first practicing UNITS, use TWO of a kind and REPEAT (8 counts).

Let's start with SINGLE RHYTHM: (One step to TWO beats of music)

COUNT: 1   2   3   4

1. Practice: "SIDE (Touch)"   "SIDE (Touch)"
   Foot Positions: 2nd   1st   2nd   1st
2. Practice: "FORWARD (Touch)"   "FORWARD (Touch)"
3. Practice: "BACK (Touch)"   "BACK (Touch)"
4. Practice: "FORWARD (Touch)"   "BACK (Touch)"
   Foot Positions: 4th   3rd   4th   3rd
5. Practice ALONE and then with a partner. MAN will always start with his LEFT FOOT. LADY will always start with her RIGHT FOOT. LADY'S PART will always be a NATURAL OPPOSITE.

NOW let's do some DOUBLE RHYTHM UNITS. The DOUBLE RHYTHM UNITS in the following patterns are all CHASSÉS. A "CHASSÉ" is a "SIDE TOGETHER," (two QUICK STEPS to TWO beats of music).

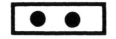 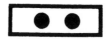

1. Practice, saying: "SIDE TOGETHER"   "SIDE TOGETHER"
2. Practice with the MAN with his BACK to the center of the room. Starting with his LEFT foot, he and his partner will travel LINE OF DANCE traveling to the man's LEFT.
3. PRACTICE the reverse by having the man start with his RIGHT FOOT, and FACING the center of the room.
4. CHASSÉ comes from the French term "to chase." The Closing foot constantly CHASSÉS the other foot.

     Let's start now with the simplest form of Foxtrot Patterns. . . . TWO UNIT PATTERNS that are composed of only ONE RHYTHM UNIT. The RHYTHM UNIT is a DOUBLE (Two steps to Two beats of music). By putting TWO DOUBLES together, we have a series of FOUR BEAT PATTERNS. . . . Each pattern will start with the man's LEFT foot free and the lady's RIGHT foot free.

     Description of the Patterns listed are for the MAN'S PARTS. (Ladies will do a "Natural Opposite" unless otherwise specified.)

     TWO UNIT PATTERNS . . . (Double Rhythm) STEP on EVERY BEAT. The patterns described in this section are recognized by several names. FOUR BEAT RHYTHM danced to SLOW lilting music is often referred to as NITECLUB FOXTROT or simply SLOW DANCING. If the music is fast, it becomes TROT RHYTHM and develops a rhythmic bounce. Practice to all tempos for versatility.

COUNT:	1	2		3	4

UNIT:	●	●		●	●

1. BASIC STEP: F   F   S   T
2. LEFT TURN: F   B   S   T   (look over OWN left shoulder to make a gradual left turn.)
3. CONVERSATION: ⎰F   F   S   T   (face each other for
    (Lady)   ⎱F   F   S   T   counts 3 & 4)
4. CHASSÉ: S   T   S   T
5. DIAGONAL BASIC: (Same as Basic step except that man steps OUTSIDE the lady in Right Parallel for counts ONE and TWO.) (Contrabody Shoulder)
6. DIAGONAL WALKS: F   F   S   T
         and B   B   S   T

     (Diagonal walks travel around LOD by angling the man's forward steps diagonal to the wall . . . and his backward steps diagonally to the center. His SIDE TOGETHER step will face the outside wall.)

COUNT:	1	2		3	4

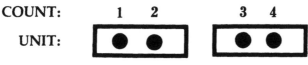

7. RIGHT TURN: B   F   S   T   (gradual Right turn)
     (Look over OWN right shoulder to aid the execution of the turn.)
8. BASIC PIVOT (LEFT)   ⎰F   F   F   B
    (Lady)   ⎱F   F ↶   B   F
     (Partners start in conversation position. Lady faces man on count 3.)
9. RIGHT PIVOT: ⎰F   F ↷   S↷F
    (Lady)   ⎱F   F   F   B
     (Lady steps between man's feet on count 3, turning Right.)

Most of the THREE UNIT PATTERNS can also be done in TWO UNITS by changing the two SINGLE RHYTHM UNITS to one DOUBLE RHYTHM UNIT. (Experiment on your own.)

THREE UNIT PATTERNS . . . referred to in most Dance Teaching Circles as BASIC RHYTHM: . . . composed of two SINGLE RHYTHM UNITS and one DOUBLE.

COUNT:	1	2		3	4		5	6
UNIT:	●	/		●	/		●	●
1. BASIC STEP:	F	(t)		F	(t)		S	T
2. CONVERSATION:	F	(t)		F	(t)		S	T
(Lady):	F	(t)		F	(t)		S	T
3. BASIC LEFT TURN:	F	(hold)		B	(t)		S	T

(The "touch" in 1st foot position is not necessary in this Left Turn . . . Man's body leans slightly back on counts ONE and TWO.)

| 4. OVERSWAY: | Side | (t) | | Side | (t) | | S | T |

- Practice the pattern ALONE . . . and then with a partner.

- Practice, thinking of the CENTER POINT OF BALANCE moving WITH the FREE FOOT while the TOP of the body stays with the WEIGHTED FOOT, on the first TWO UNITS of the pattern. (This action produces the SWAY in the OVERSWAY.)

- Practice, emphasizing the PRESS into the floor of the weighted foot on the AND before each unit.

- Practice, thinking of FOOTWORK. Remember that all SIDE steps land on the ball of the foot before lowering to the flat foot.

5. WALK THRU:

COUNT:	1	2	3	4	5	6
UNIT:	●	/	●	/	●	●
BOTH Say:	"SIDE Touch		SIDE Touch		WALK THRU"	
Man's Direction:	Side LEFT		Side RIGHT		FORWARD FORWARD	
Lady's Direction:	Side RIGHT		Side LEFT		FORWARD FORWARD	
DANCE POSITION:	CLOSED		CLOSED		*CONVERSATION	

- *CONVERSATION POSITION means that BOTH partners form a V shape with the Lady's LEFT hip in contact with the MAN'S RIGHT HIP. BOTH partners will move FORWARD to the MAN'S Left.

- Practice this pattern, starting with the man's BACK to the center of the room. Both partners will then be traveling around the room counter-clockwise or LINE OF DANCE (LOD).

- Practice alternating an OVERSWAY with a WALK THRU before going on to the next step.

- Practice, thinking of the CENTER POINT OF BALANCE. Note that an EXTRA push is needed on the AND count before the last UNIT. The MAN gives EXTRA EMPHASIS to count 5 and coasts thru count 6.

6. **DIAGONAL BASIC:** (Same as Basic Step except that man steps OUTSIDE Lady in Right Parallel position for counts ONE, brush two, and THREE, brush four.)

7. **DIAGONAL WALKS:** (Same as Diagonal walks in TWO UNIT pattern except that the Forward and Backward steps are SINGLE RHYTHM instead of Double.)

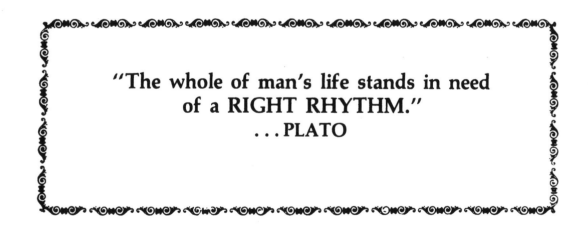

	F	(t)	F	(t)	S	T
and	B	(t)	B	(t)	S	T
8. OPEN LEFT CROSS TURN:	F	(hold)	↓B	(t)	S	F
(Lady):	B	(hold)	F	(t)	F	F
9. BASIC RIGHT TURN:	B	(hold)	F	(t)	S	T
10. CONVERSATION PIVOT:	‹F	(t)	F	(t)↓	B	F
(Right Pivot)						
11. CONVERSATION PIVOT:	‹F	(t)	F	(t)	↓F	↓B
(Left Pivot)						
(Lady):	‹F	(t)	F	↓(t)	B	F

> "The whole of man's life stands in need
> of a RIGHT RHYTHM."
> ...PLATO

87

Teachers of Dance: Please read TEACHERS NOTE on the last page of Foxtrot, before teaching FOUR UNIT PATTERNS.

FOUR UNIT PATTERNS, alternating DOUBLE and SINGLE RHYTHM are called BOX RHYTHM.

COUNT:	1	2		3	4		5	6		7	8

UNIT: (● ●) (● /) (● ●) (● /)

1. SIDE BASIC: S   T   S   (t)   S   T   S   (t)

(Use the action of an OVERSWAY on all SINGLE RHYTHM SIDE steps.)

2. LEFT BOX
TURN: Side Tog.   Fwd. (t)   Side Tog.   Back (t)

(Both partners look LEFT and let the body gradually turn left.)

• Practice facing one direction just long enough to discover the four CORNERS of the "BOX" step.

• Practice turning slightly LEFT by looking over your OWN LEFT shoulder as you do the pattern.

• Practice emphasizing the MAN'S STEP FORWARD in 4th foot position BETWEEN the lady's feet on count 3.

• Practice emphasizing the LADY'S STEP FORWARD in 4th foot position BETWEEN the man's feet on count 7.

• Practice stepping HEEL FIRST on all of the FORWARD steps (HEEL, meaning the FLAT of the heel). (The SIDE TOGETHER steps will be taken with the heel slightly OFF the floor.)

• Practice your TURNING BOX STEP until you can do a complete turn (returning to LINE OF DANCE) in 16 counts of music (Eight UNITS, or TWO complete BOX STEPS).

• Practice thinking DRIVE with the CENTER POINT OF BALANCE on the FIRST BEAT of every UNIT. The CENTER POINT OF BALANCE will be DRIVING in the direction of the moving foot.

3. TRAVELING BOX: S   T   F   (t)   S   T   F   (t)

(Shoulders will alternate from being on a Right diagonal to being on a Left diagonal on count THREE and return to Right diagonal on count SEVEN.) (See Contra Body Movement.)

4. SINGLE TWINKLE: S   T   F   (t)   S   T   F   (t)
(Lady):   S   T   B   S   T   F

("Twinkle" occurs on count SIX, placing partners in conversation position.)

5. FALLAWAY CHECK: B   T   F   (hold)   B   T   F   (t)
(Lady):   B   T   F   (hold)   B   T   F   (t)

(Partners start in closed position. Man leads Lady to step, crossing behind her own foot on count ONE, producing a SWIVEL on count TWO and a CHECK, in Right Parallel position on count THREE.

88

6. SPIRAL: S   T   F   (t)   S   T   F   (t)

(Man alternates Left and Right Parallel positions on each FORWARD step. This produces a zig-zag pattern as it travels around LOD.)

7. BOX SPIN TURN: S   T   B↓   F   B   B

(Precede with a RIGHT turn to start pattern with man backing LOD.)

8. OPEN LEFT BOX TURN: S   F   F   S   B   B

(Can be danced in CLOSED position or in Parallel.)

9. BOX RHYTHM PIVOTS: B↓   F↓   B↓   F↓   B↓   F↓

(Right Pivots) (Precede with any RIGHT TURN. For contrast try exiting with a Left Turn.)

10. BOX RHYTHM PIVOTS: F↰   B↰   F↰   B↰   F↰   B↰

(Left Pivots) (Precede with Conversation Walks . . . two SINGLES, walking in conversation position. Lady turns Left to start Pivots.)

MIXED RHYTHMS are easy, once you have mastered the various combinations. It is suggested that you practice patterns in each category, STAYING WITH ONE RHYTHM until it becomes comfortable and you understand the patterns you are doing.

The NEXT STEP is to find that ANY COMBINATION is possible by selecting "one of these . . . and one of those." Here are a few MIXED RHYTHMS to start you out . . .

COUNT:	1 2	3 4	5 6	7 8	1 2	3 4	5 6	7 8
UNIT:	● /	● /	● ●	● /	● ●	● ●	● ●	●
	F (t)	F (t)	S T	S (t)	B S	F S	B S	F

GRAPEVINE:

(The KEY UNIT is on count ONE of the 2nd set of EIGHT. Man leads girl into RIGHT PARALLEL position to start the GRAPEVINE.)

ADVANCED RHYTHM PROGRESSIONS:

Without even seeing the Units in terms of DOTS, let's try a pattern with just the Annotation symbols: F=Forward, B=Back etc. The symbols will be SPACED in UNITS. . . .

SLOW TROT:

F	F	S T	F	F	F	S T	F

(16 beats of music.)

SYNCOPATED LOCK:

F	S T	F	F Hk F

(This leaves man's RIGHT foot free. It is suggested that you follow this pattern with another Syncopated Lock to finish with the man's LEFT foot free. The TRIPLE in this pattern is merely a basic RHYTHM VARIATION of a SINGLE RHYTHM UNIT.)

89

ONE UNIT "LINKS" . . . To join other patterns together to make them "flow" or to make them PHRASE to the Music . . . or to return to a different free foot.

1. WALKING STEPS . . . (Forward or Backward Steps in SINGLE RHYTHM.)

2. TROTTING STEPS . . . (Forward or Backward DOUBLE RHYTHM UNITS.)

3. CHASSÉ'S . . . ("Side Together" DOUBLE RHYTHM steps.)

4. CHECKS . . . (a DOUBLE RHYTHM UNIT stepping FORWARD and then BACK.)

5. OVERSWAYS . . . (alternating SIDE STEPS to SINGLE RHYTHM.)

6. PIVOTS . . . (DOUBLE RHYTHM or SINGLE RHYTHM turning either Left or Right in 4th Foot Position.)

LEADING FOXTROT we have a choice of CLOSED BODY CONTACT or partners several inches apart, but in closed dancing position. For Basic SOCIAL DANCING, we suggest that the latter is easier to teach and more comfortable for the average person. The resistance that is desired is achieved in TWO ways. The Man's hand "cradles" the Lady's back, just below her left shoulder blade and slightly toward center. Her Left hand is behind his Right shoulder with arms lightly touching. His shoulder will press into her hand, completing the circular resistance. (See pictures of Dance Positions. . . .)

TEACHERS NOTE: No doubt that many teachers will wonder WHY start the Box Rhythm Patterns with the DOUBLE RHYTHM instead of the SINGLE. This was the result of several years of experimentation. You will find that your students will no longer "Foxtrot their Waltz . . . or Waltz their Foxtrot" if you use the prescribed approach. Also, the teaching of a SINGLE TWINKLE and particularly of an OPEN LEFT BOX becomes an easy matter when you START with the SIDE step. Many of your OLD FAVORITES will take on a new look, just by rearranging their starting point. Give it a try.

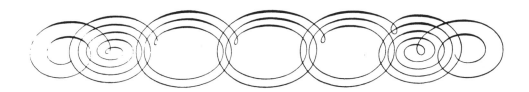

TANGO

Tango is one of the most fascinating of all the dances. The control it develops is unmatched in any other dance. A GOOD TANGO DANCER can lead or follow anyone. With a little altering of rhythm, the patterns are interchangeable with Fox Trot, and with Contemporary Tango Hustle.

For exhibition dancing, a Tango dancer must develop a strong connection with the music, the dance, and the audience. The audience can only "feel" this connection if the performer feels and projects this feeling. So it is when dancing for your own pleasure — and your partner's!!

Styles vary in Tango: Argentine, French, Gaucho and International. Still, Tango has become one of our American "Standards" regardless of its origin. The Americanized version is a combination of the best parts of each. The principals involved are the same for ANY good dancing. First, the dance must fit the MUSIC. Second, it must contain the basic CHARACTERISTICS that set it apart from other dances. Third, it must be comfortable and pleasing to do — and above all — IT MUST NOT LOOK DATED!!

In Tango, slightly flexed knees (not noticeably bent) are a "must." This settles the weight in the lower part of the body and gives you a feeling of closeness to the ground. (Direct opposite of Waltz where one feels lifted.)

On occasion, a girl will find herself in a position of having to follow Tango with someone whose style she does not know. A good rule is to stay with the man's RIGHT thigh. Assuming that he is a good dancer, you will be able to imagine a magnet in HIS RIGHT and YOUR LEFT thigh. Even when you are led into open position, you will snap back for the close when the pattern is completed.

PHRASING is an important part of Tango. You will notice that all of the basic patterns are eight beat patterns. By starting at the beginning of a phrase and doing an EVEN number of 8 beat patterns, you will stay on phrase. We call this "automatic phrasing." Most Tango music phrases to 16 or 32 beats of music. Tango music is like a story. It contains paragraphs, (MAJOR PHRASES); sentences (MINOR PHRASES); and the period at the end of each sentence is the "Tango Close."

TANGO CLOSE: The Tango close is a Double and a Blank Unit that ends each basic pattern. Unless otherwise specified, "Tango close" will refer to a basic "Forward-Side-Touch and Hold."

BASIC TECHNIQUE: The difference in basic technique of Tango from Foxtrot, lies in the actual point at which one foot passes the other. In a SINGLE RHYTHM (slow) count in Foxtrot, the foot brushes or "follows thru" on the 2nd count. In Tango, the brush does not come until AFTER the 2nd count. Thus we count Tango 1 2 & 3 4 & — The BRUSH occurring on the "&" count.

In the FORWARD STEPS in Tango, the FREE FOOT stays behind for the second beat of the UNIT. However, the BODY (CPB) continues to move FORWARD. This requires practice.

Example:

	1	2	&		3	4	&
	●		/		●		/

FOOT DIRECTION: Forward & Hold   Forward & Hold
CPB: F   F   F   F

Practice these FORWARD moves by themselves. Then practice the TANGO CLOSE by itself. The TANGO CLOSE is a DOUBLE [● ●] and a BLANK [/] .

Note the description of the SHOULDER PULL on counts 5 and 6. Then proceed with the patterns.

1. BASIC STEP . . .

COUNT:	1 2 &	3 4 &	5 6	7 8
UNIT:	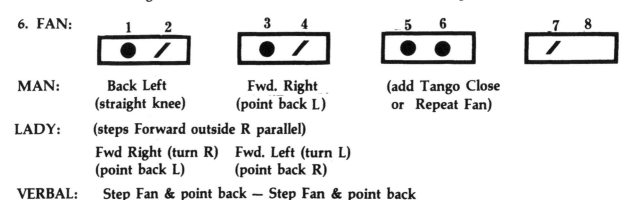			
FOOT:	LEFT	RIGHT	L R	
Direction:	"Forward	Forward	Frwd. Side	(touch) (hold)"
Shoulder Pull:	Back Left	Back Right	Bk. L. Bk. R.	Neutral

(LADY steps natural opposite.)

2. OUTSIDE PARALLEL . . .

Same COUNT and same PATTERN as above, except that the man steps OUTSIDE the LADY in RIGHT PARALLEL on counts ONE hold two . . . and THREE hold four. Shoulders on a RIGHT Diagonal, RIGHT shoulder back. (1,2,3,4.) Finish with "Tango Close" as above.

3. SLOW CHANGE . . .

MAN: "Forward (point back)   Back (point Fwd.)   Back Side   (touch) (hold)"

LADY: Back   FORWARD   FORWARD Side   (touch) (hold)
(moving toward RIGHT Parallel, Finish in
CONVERSATION.) both partners facing L.O.D.

4. CONVERSATION . . .

MAN: <   "Forward   Forward   &   Frwd. Side   (touch) (hold)"

LADY: <   Forward   Forward (turn L) BACK Side   (touch) (hold)

5. DIP:

	1	2	3	4	5-6-7-8
(CORTE') MAN:	DIP Back Left		RETURN Forward Right		(add a TANGO CLOSE or)
	Bent LEFT knee		(straight LEFT Knee)		(just REPEAT the DIP)

On the DIP . . . Both partners center their weight over the WEIGHTED FOOT. Practice doing each pattern ALONE. Each supports his OWN weight. Shoulders should be angled with RIGHT SHOULDER BACK on the Dip.

6. FAN:

1 2	3 4	5 6	7 8

MAN: Back Left   Fwd. Right   (add Tango Close
        (straight knee) (point back L)   or Repeat Fan)

LADY: (steps Forward outside R parallel)

Fwd Right (turn R)   Fwd. Left (turn L)
(point back L)   (point back R)

VERBAL: Step Fan & point back — Step Fan & point back
                1   2   3   4

92

7. OPEN FAN (16 beat pattern) (count 2 sets of 8)

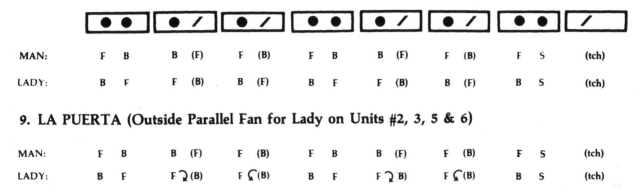

MAN:	F		F		F	S	(T) hold		F	↶	F	(B)	F	S	(T) hold
LADY:	F		F	↶	B	S	(T) hold		F	↷	F	↶	B	S	(T) hold

8. MEDIO CORTE' (DIP on 2nd. & 4th. UNITS)

MAN:	F	B	B	(F)	F	(B)	F	B	B	(F)	F	(B)	F	S	(tch)
LADY:	B	F	F	(B)	B	(F)	B	F	F	(B)	B	(F)	B	S	(tch)

9. LA PUERTA (Outside Parallel Fan for Lady on Units #2, 3, 5 & 6)

MAN:	F	B	B	(F)	F	(B)	F	B	B	(F)	F	(B)	F	S	(tch)
LADY:	B	F	F ↷	(B)	F ↶	(B)	B	F	F ↷	B)	F ↶	(B)	B	S	(tch)

Most of the TANGO emphasizes CONTRA-BODY MOVEMENT. Practice the individual patterns thinking first of FOOT POSITION . . . and then of SHOULDERS.

10. LA PUERTA with DIP (TWO Rocking Steps Precede the FAN. NO Rocking Steps between the FAN and the DIP. Total count is TWO SETS of EIGHT.) (16 beats)

COUNT:	1	2	3	4	5	6	7	8	1	2	3	4	5	6	7	8
	F	B	F	B	B(hold)	F(hold)	B	(f)	F	(b)	F	S	(t) hold
					(Fan Girl)	(Return)	DIP		(Return)		TANGO CLOSE		

11. Time to try some RHYTHM VARIATIONS. Go back to Pattern #2. OUTSIDE PARALLEL. Keep the same DIAGONAL POSITION (Right shoulder pulled back) and replace the first UNIT with a TRIPLE ("side together side"). Second Unit will step FORWARD, still outside Right Parallel and complete the pattern as usual. (See REPRINT next page.)

Replace the first Unit of Step #4. CONVERSATION. ONE TRIPLE, "SIDE TOGETHER SIDE" . . . then BOTH step FORWARD with the INSIDE FOOT & complete the pattern.

12. We can use LINKS to get back in time with the music . . . or to make a particular piece of music PHRASE. Not ALL Tango Music phrases to sets of eight. Practice QUICK LEFT TURNS: "FORWARD BACK SIDE TOGETHER," turning Left. TWO of those would make an eight beat pattern. ONE would make a TWO UNIT LINK and EITHER of the DOUBLE RHYTHM UNITS (FORWARD BACK . . . or . . . SIDE TOGETHER) would make a ONE UNIT LINK. Practice putting QUICK LEFT TURNS in between other patterns. Always use a complete set of EIGHT counts unless the music calls for less.

13. For Advanced students, try some of the SYNCOPATIONS using the following guide.

TANGO CLOSE:

Basic:	FORWARD SIDE	(TOUCH HOLD)
UNIT:	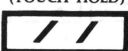	

Syncopated:	FORWARD SIDE	TOGETHER SIDE (HOLD)
COUNT:	5 6	and 7 (8)
UNIT:		

(A BLANK UNIT is interchangeable with a DOUBLE RHYTHM UNIT. It could be a PRIMARY DOUBLE or a SYNCOPATED DOUBLE.)

14. One last idea for Advanced Students. Think of TANGO as a SERIES of RHYTHM UNITS. Now REARRANGE the UNITS to form another RHYTHM PATTERN. See how many variations you can create on your own.

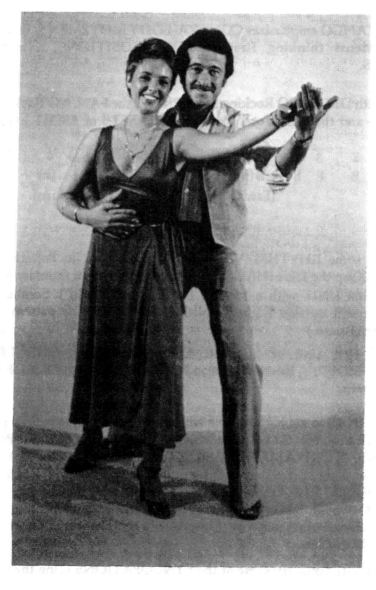

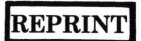
Reprint from Dance Views Publications, June 1975

We have had requests for more BASIC VARIATIONS in ARGENTINE TANGO. Here are 3 more that are out of the new GOLDEN STATE CURRICULUM.

A simple but effective variation in BASIC ARGENTINE TANGO: (We present TWO variations from the same basic step by simply substituting one RHYTHM UNIT for another.)

This BASIC PATTERN is a SLOW CHANGE. Directions are for the man. Pattern starts in closed position . . . girl steps OUTSIDE man on count 5. Pattern ends in conversation position.

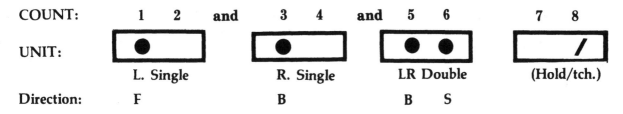

COUNT:	1	2	and	3	4	and	5	6		7	8
UNIT:	L. Single			R. Single			LR Double			(Hold/tch.)	
Direction:	F			B			B	S			

Now, from conversation position, BOTH partners do a "SIDE TOGETHER SIDE" on counts 1&2. BOTH partners step thru (Forward) on count 3. Close the position for the TANGO CLOSE.

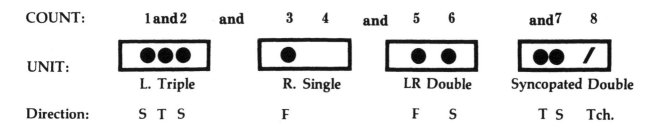

COUNT:	1 and 2	and	3	4	and	5	6		7	8
UNIT:	L. Triple		R. Single			LR Double			(Hold/or tch.)	
Direction:	S T S		F			F	S			

We can further develop this same pattern by "syncopating" the "TANGO CLOSE" (the last two Units of the pattern). Instead of "holding" the counts of 7 and 8, we actually STEP again on the "and" and on the "8":

COUNT:	1 and 2	and	3	4	and	5	6	and 7	8
UNIT:	L. Triple		R. Single			LR Double		Syncopated Double	
Direction:	S T S		F			F	S	T S	Tch.

S=Side/ T=Together/ F=Forward/ Tch=Touch/ ● =a STEP or "Wt. Change" S=Side

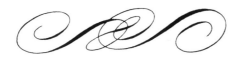

...SAMBA...

SAMBA is a "FUN DANCE" — it is also a great exercise for developing flexibility. Samba is often referred to as Brazilian Waltz. Many of the patterns are interchangeable with our own Viennese Waltz.

The BASIC CHARACTERISTIC of Samba is the lilting bounce. Once the basic bouncing movement is developed, it becomes more subtle and more a "feeling" of bounce than actually being able to see it.

There are TWO basic movements to Samba. One counteracts the other. Flexible knees produce the BOUNCE — PENDULUM motion swings the body forward and back, taking up the SLACK; thus making the bounce more "felt" than seen.

In Samba, it is extremely important to keep the midriff firm, head tall, shoulders comfortably erect.

Before attempting patterns, practice the basic movement. With both feet together (1st foot position), relax and bounce, sinking (bouncing down) on every count. The rise is on the "and" between the counts:

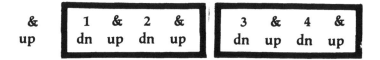

&		1	&	2	&		3	&	4	&
up		dn	up	dn	up		dn	up	dn	up

Next ... try shifting weight on EVERY UNIT in 4th foot position:

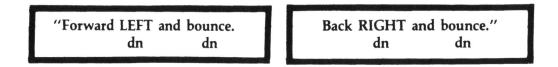

"Forward LEFT and bounce.		Back RIGHT and bounce."
dn dn		dn dn

Now, let's get on to the actual patterns. Note as you go through them, how many patterns are similar to other dances. Samba not only teaches FLEXIBILITY, but also quick CHANGES of WEIGHT and quick changes of DIRECTION.

On a CONTEMPORARY NOTE ... Those who were familiar with SAMBA were able to use some of the movements and patterns in SOLO ROCK routines ... and then later in the various forms of HUSTLE. The BASICS of SAMBA are important for the development of EVERY DANCE!

SAMBA

... Man will always start with his LEFT FOOT ... Lady with the RIGHT. (Standard Ballroom Closed Position hold for LATIN)

1. CAIXO ... (pronounced Kigh. . .ee. . .she. . .oh) The Caixo is merely a long narrow BOX STEP. The "side togethers" are very small (particularly when the music is fast).

COUNT:	1 & a 2	and	3 & a 4
UNIT:	● ●●		● ●●
MAN:	Fwd. Side Tog.		Back Side Tog.
LADY:	Back Side Tog.		Fwd. Side Tog.

(entire pattern is a gradual LEFT TURN.)
BOTH partners look over their OWN Left shoulder.

2. BALANCETE ... Side Balance steps, stepping in 5th foot position with very little weight on the "a" count. Resist the temptation to step on the "and" count. Delay the "and" and step on the "a."

COUNT:	1 & a 2	and	3 & a 4
UNIT	● ●●		● ●●
BOTH:	Side 5th Place		Side 5th Place
Foot Pos.:	2nd 5th 5th		2nd/5th 5th
Basic Movement:	Down & Down	up	Down & Down

3. COPA ... Both partners are traveling forward together in CONVERSATION POSITION (precede a COPA with two BALANCETES).

The COPA is a FOUR UNIT PATTERN ... Both partners traveling forward

COUNT:	1 & a 2	3 & a 4
UNIT:	● ●●	● ●●
BOTH:	Frwd.	Frwd.

Repeat for a 3rd UNIT and then CLOSE facing each other on 7 & 8.

The FOOTWORK "CALL" throughout is "FLAT and TOE FLAT" with very little weight on the BALL OF THE FOOT for the "toe" count.

4. REVERSE COPA: 4 unit pattern — consisting of one Balancete and 3 Copas. The three Copas change direction — alternating one Copa facing LOD, and the next toward your partner.

Man's "Verbal" pattern:	L Balancete	R Copa	L Copa	R Copa
Partners facing:	each other	away	each other	away
Man's L hand leads:	Left	forward	back	forward

(Lady natural opposite.)

5. DOUBLE COPA: A Reverse Copa (4 units) followed by a straight Copa produces a Double Copa. The change of direction occurs on the 1st unit of the Straight Copa. (Fwd. L on count 1 & turn L to reverse direction.)

6. RITMO: a "marking time" or "rest" step ... particularly helpful as a preparation for other patterns. Lilting, subtle bounce of "Down Down."

COUNT:	1 & a 2		3 & a 4	
MAN:	PL.	S PL.	PL.	S PL.
FOOT POS.:	1st	2nd 2nd	1st	2nd 2nd

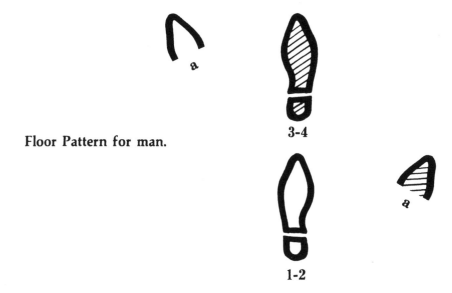

1-2   3-4

7. PAULISTA: a "traveling" Ritmo for the man ... a "traveling" Balancete for the girl. Man progresses forward ... girl backward. Man changes weight on every unit, with the free foot pointing directly side (2nd foot position). This produces a "gripping" action in order to change the girl from side to side on every "&" count.

Floor Pattern for man.

3-4

1-2

8. BRAZILIAN CAIXO: — Merely an extension of the regular caixo, the Brazilian adds a new motion ... a CIRCULAR motion. Our "pendulum" not only swings back and forth, but now swings into a circle. (Keep turning Left.)

All the way thru Samba, we find that the motion produces a "Flat — toe — Flat," or shifting of complete weight on every unit. The farther we progress, the more important this element becomes.

COUNT:	1 & a 2	&	3 & a 4	
MAN:	F	S X	B	S T
ʼADY:	B	S T	F	S X

9. SAMBA WALKS — lilting strides

COUNT:	1	2		3 & a 4			5	6		7 & a 8		
	●	●		●	● ●		●	●		●	● ●	
FOOT:	F	F		F	S	T	F	F		F	S	T
Shoulder	L	R		L	R	L	R	L		R	L	R
PULL:	L	R		L			R	L		R		

QUIZ:

1. What is the Basic Movement Unit in Samba ? _____

2. On which counts of the triple do we step?
   _____   _____   _____

3. Can all three Primary Rhythm Units be danced in Samba ? _____

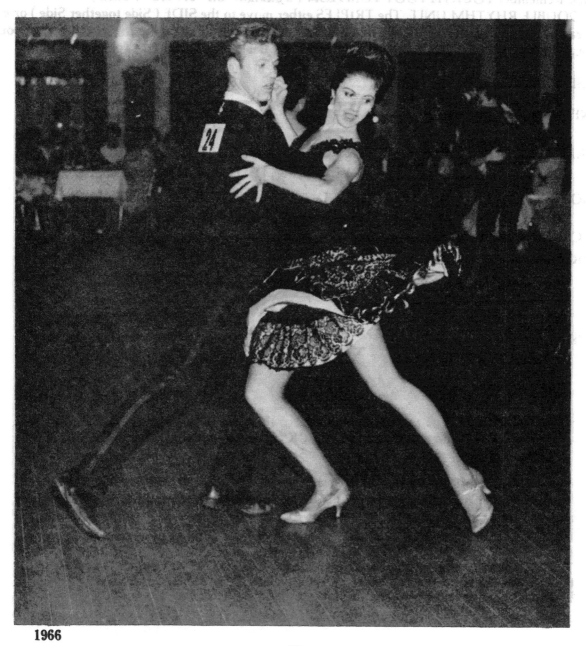

1966

CHA CHA

CHA CHA is a FOUR UNIT PATTERN alternating DOUBLE and TRIPLE RHYTHM UNITS. That simply means that you "STEP TWICE" and "STEP THREE TIMES" and "STEP TWICE" and "STEP THREE TIMES." Popularized in the 50's, Cha Cha has become an American STANDARD. Actually, the Cha Cha was an outgrowth of MAMBO. Mambo was a Dancer's dance and required too much dance education to become popular with the average social dancer. Cha Cha slowed down the tempo and made the dance easier to learn.

Practice the individual UNITS without music before dancing the patterns to music. In Cha Cha the DOUBLE RHYTHM UNITS are referred to as "Breaks." A "Break" in Cha Cha is a "Change of direction." The first STEP of the Unit is either FORWARD, or BACKWARD. The Second STEP of the DOUBLE RHYTHM UNIT returns to its original position.

Please note that the DIRECTION refers to the CENTER POINT OF BALANCE (CPB) as well as the foot placement. Therefore to step FORWARD and then return to the back foot, the annotation would read F B for "Forward . . . Back"

The FOOT POSITION for the BREAKS remains the same for all of the basic patterns. Remember FOURTH FOOT POSITION (a straight line forward or back) when dancing the DOUBLE RHYTHM UNIT. The TRIPLES either move to the SIDE (Side together Side) or in a straight line (run run run). Everything else is just a matter of changing the direction that you face. Man starts with LEFT foot free . . . Lady with her RIGHT foot free for each pattern.

1. SIDE BASIC:

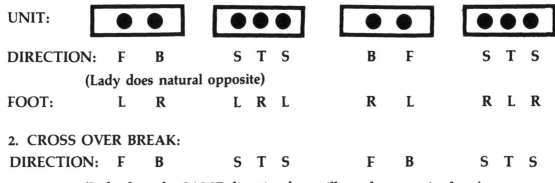

UNIT:												
DIRECTION:	F	B		S	T	S		B	F		S	T	S
FOOT:	L	R		L	R	L		R	L		R	L	R

(Lady does natural opposite)

2. CROSS OVER BREAK:

DIRECTION:	F	B		S	T	S		F	B		S	T	S

(Lady does the SAME direction but still on the opposite foot.)

POSITION:

- BOTH partners do a "FORWARD BACK" to the man's RIGHT WALL (inside foot please)
- Face each other for the TRIPLE
- BOTH do a "Forward Back" to the man's LEFT wall (start with inside foot again)
- Finish the last TRIPLE facing each other as you started.

The lead consists of releasing one hand for each CROSSOVER. Contact is maintained with the hand that is closest to your partner (the INSIDE HAND.) The hand change takes place on the last step of the TRIPLE.

3. BREAK TURN: (precede with a CrossOver Break)

The man starts his CROSSOVER BREAK to his RIGHT side when his LEFT foot is free. He starts the BREAK TURN to his LEFT side when his RIGHT foot is free.

UNIT:

VERBAL: "Cross to the RIGHT & Cha Cha Cha . . . Break turn LEFT & Cha Cha Cha."

POSITION:

4. PROGRESSIVE BASIC:

UNIT:

DIRECTION: F   B   B   B   B   B   F   F   F   F

5. CROSS BODY LEAD:

SHE: B   F   F   F   F   F (½ B   S   T   S

HE: F   B (¼   S   T   S   B (¼ F   S   T   S

POSITIONS:

6. DOUBLE CROSS OVER:

To do a DOUBLE CROSS OVER just repeat the BREAK STEP on each side of a CROSS OVER BREAK. Man leads by keeping his partner's hand extended to each wall for the "BREAK STEP and BREAK STEP."

This pattern can be repeated as many times as you wish EXCEPT that you must do a DOUBLE BREAK an EVEN number of times to put you back on phrase with the music.

7. PARALLEL BREAKS:

Dance a SIDE BASIC but substitute LEFT and RIGHT PARALLEL BREAKS . . . Man does all FORWARD Breaks and SHE does all BACK Breaks. The Cha Cha Cha in between is a little "Side Together Side."

UNIT:

POSITIONS:

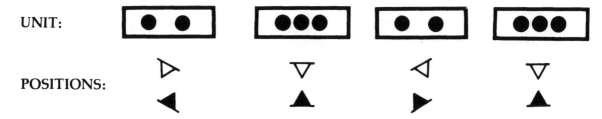

8. SWEETHEART:

Dance a SIDE BASIC or a PROGRESSIVE BASIC and switch to HANDSHAKE PO-SITION on the man's FORWARD BREAK. On the TRIPLE place the girl to the man's RIGHT SIDE. (see Butterfly position in Latin Hustle.)

BOTH partners do a BACK BREAK with lady on man's RIGHT side and then with the lady on the man's LEFT side. Once more on his RIGHT side and then return her to her original position in front of her partner.

9. WHEEL:

Dance the FIRST TWO UNITS of a CROSS BODY LEAD. This places the lady in a right CORNER POSITION with her LEFT foot free. HE is to her LEFT with his RIGHT foot free.

The man pulls his LEFT shoulder back sharply to start walking BACKWARD maintaining the RHYTHM PATTERN of the Cha Cha. This action propels the girl FORWARD and the two partners revolve around an imaginary pole to produce a WHEEL.

The WHEEL itself is composed of FOUR UNITS traveling in the circle.

The EXIT from the Wheel completes the phrase with TWO MORE UNITS: As the Wheel ends, SHE is on the man's RIGHT side.

SHE:	↶F⤸	B	F	F	F
HE:	B	F	F	F	F

SHE PIVOTS in front of him . . . to place herself on the man's LEFT SIDE . . . BOTH travel forward on the TRIPLE . . . finish pattern with a CROSSOVER BREAK.

10. RHYTHM VARIATIONS:

MAMBO can be danced by substituting SINGLE RHYTHM for every TRIPLE in the Cha Cha. Practice each pattern dancing a "STEP HOLD" instead of a "Cha Cha Cha." That will get you started. Next, SPEED up the music . . . gradually you will work your way up to a MAMBO TEMPO.

Refer to ADVANCED SYNCOPATION UNITS and try all of the varieties that can be substituted for DOUBLE RHYTHM. You will be amazed! Your "BREAK STEP" can become a "KICK BREAK STEP."

A really smooth RHYTHM VARIATION can be danced in either CHA CHA or MAMBO by dancing a DELAYED SINGLE instead of the TRIPLE. Say, "LIFT STEP" or "KICK STEP" instead of "STEP THREE TIMES."

11. STYLE VARIATIONS and PATTERN VARIATIONS are unlimited.

Refer to the Dance Positions in some of the contemporary dances . . . (Cradle, Macho, Pretzel etc.) . . . now dance a BASIC CHA CHA pattern holding TWO HAND POSITION. Maintain the CHA CHA BEAT and move from one position to another . . . FANTASTIC!

DANCING TO THE MUSIC ...

To quote one of the all time great MAMBO DANCERS of our time, "If you can't dance CHA CHA on the TWO BEAT ... DON'T BOTHER DANCING CHA CHA!" ROCKI MARI, master Latin Dancer from California and Phoenix, Arizona, spends a great deal of time training dancers to hear and feel "THE TWO BEAT."

I agree with Rocki's statement completely. No reference has been made so far to dancing to CHA CHA MUSIC. Those of you who have danced FOXTROT or SWING or WALTZ would probably feel very uncomfortable if you did not start dancing on a DOWNBEAT. Many times a new dancer is not aware WHAT is wrong ... but is aware that SOMETHING is wrong when they are on the wrong beat of the music.

In CHA CHA or MAMBO or the new SALSA SUAVE ... and even in OPEN RUMBA, the dancer dances with the BODY on the DOWNBEAT but actually STEPS or BREAKS on the UPBEAT. To accomplish this, try the following exercise:

- LISTEN to ANY MUSIC that is 4/4 time. (even a MARCH) You will probably be able to pick out the ONE count. If you can hear the ONE ... you can find the TWO. It FOLLOWS the ONE!

- Pick up the end of a count of eight saying, "five six seven eight." On count ONE ... LIFT the body as if someone had punched the solar plexus (CPB) and lifted you upward ... then STEP (BREAK FORWARD) on count TWO.

- Your pattern will consist of EIGHT BEATS, but by starting on the TWO, you will be dancing to INVERTED UNITS. Try a SIDE BASIC PATTERN using the count: "2 3 — 4 & 5 — 6 7 — 8 & 1" The "2 3" will be the man's FORWARD BREAK and the "6 7" will be his BACK BREAK.

TEACHERS OF DANCE: Please note ... Teaching students to BREAK ON TWO is very important if there is ANY possibility that they might go on into competition or exhibition dancing ... or even to become an intermediate social dancer. Trying to learn it later ... after he has practiced breaking on "ONE" becomes a real chore.

Once a dancer has become educated to the TWO BEAT, it is just as uncomfortable to dance the LATIN DANCES on the DOWNBEAT ... as it is to dance FOXTROT or SWING on the UPBEAT. For ROUND DANCING some of the Cha Cha sequences break on ONE, but that is a different feeling entirely. You will be well rewarded by the FEELING that will be transmitted to your students ... if you take a little time to learn and TEACH the "BREAK ON TWO."

Dancing IN TIME to music is a MUST ...
Dancing IN PHRASE with the music is a JOY ...
But to feel the BODY RESPOND TO THE INTERPRETATION of the music...
...is ecstatic!

QUIZ:

1. How many Units in a Basic Step in CHA CHA ?_____

2. The educated beat requires breaking on which beat of the music ? _____

3. To change Cha Cha to Mambo, we can substitute which RHYTHM UNIT for the TRIPLE ? _____

4. Each UNIT contains one DOWNBEAT and one UPBEAT. In an INVERTED UNIT, which comes first ? _____

5. Each of the BREAKS listed are in which foot position ? _____

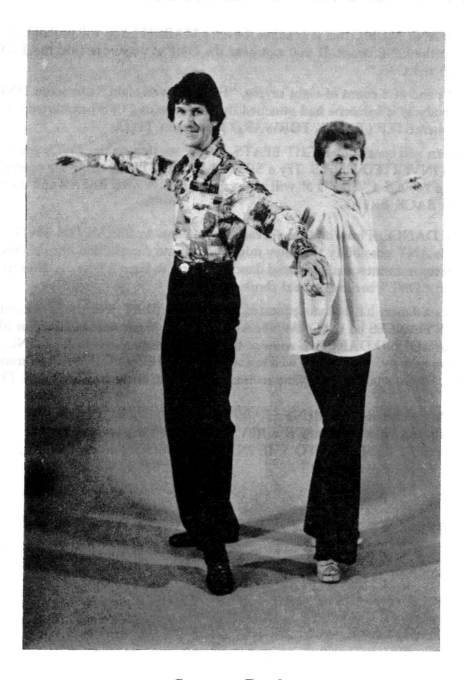

Crossover Break

CHA CHA or TANGO HUSTLE ???
1970 . . . or . . . 1978 ?

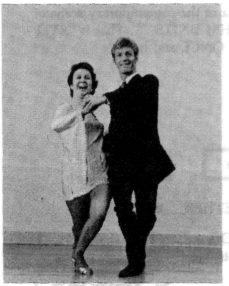

COUNT 2

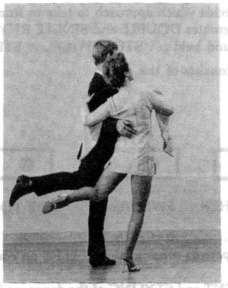

COUNT 3

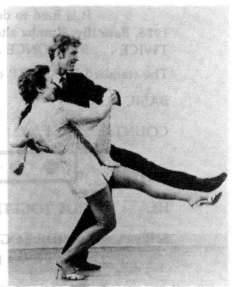

COUNT 4

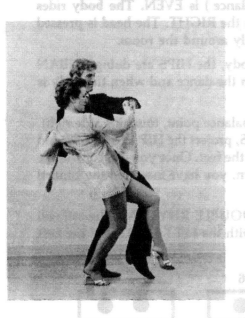

ALMOST to 5

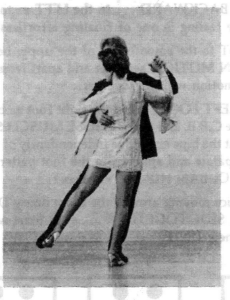

COUNT 6

• These pictures were taken in 1970 of LARRY KERN and SKIPPY BLAIR doing a ROLLER COASTER in CHA CHA. . . . OMIT that first picture & do a SYNCOPATED DOUBLE (STEP point STEP point) . . . Now start with the 2nd picture as count FOUR . . . continue as shown & add a HOOK TRIPLE at the end. (Still a great step.) (HOOK TRIPLE is the 8 & 1)

• NOW look at the pictures as TANGO HUSTLE. Start in Conversation position & step forward on ONE. Do counts 2 . . . 3 . . . 4 as shown. STEP on that forward foot on FIVE . . . STRETCH that SIX and still add the HOOK TRIPLE for 7 & 8.

Remember to keep the ESSENCE of each individual dance.

TANGO HUSTLE

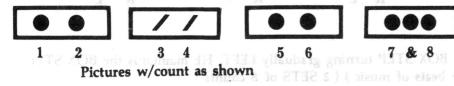

Pictures w/count as shown

CHA CHA

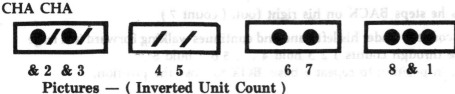

Pictures — (Inverted Unit Count)

RUMBA

It is hard to decide which approach to take to Rumba in the contemporary scene of 1978. Basically, Rumba alternates DOUBLE and SINGLE RHYTHM UNITS . . . That is "STEP TWICE . . . STEP ONCE and hold . . . STEP TWICE . . . STEP ONCE and hold."

The standard BOX STEP consists of the

BASIC BOX

COUNT:	1 2	3 4	5 6	7 8
UNIT:	[● ●]	[●]	[● ●]	[●]
HE:	"SIDE TOGETHER	FWD. (hold)	SIDE TOGETHER	BACK (hold)"
SHE:	"SIDE TOG.	BACK (hold)	SIDE TOG.	FWD. (hold) "

(entire pattern turns gradually LEFT on counts 3 and 7)

The MOVEMENT and STYLING of the dance are interwoven. The MOVEMENT of the upper body, and therefore the C.P.B. (center point of balance) is EVEN. The body rides smoothly FORWARD . . . BACKWARD . . . to the LEFT or to the RIGHT. The head is pressed upward the ceiling and the feeling is one of floating effortlessly around the room.

In CONTRAST to the smoothness of the upper body, the HIPS are doing CUBAN MOTION. Practice CUBAN MOTION separate and apart from the dance and when the body is ready, the dance and the motion will get together.

Stand on the LEFT FOOT, using the right foot as balance point, touching side right. Now find the muscles in the C.P.B. and using THOSE MUSCLES, project the HIP to the LEFT and to the RIGHT. Find out that the hips can move independently of the feet. Once you can control the movement of the HIPS, separate and apart from the foot pattern, you have mastered the control that is necessary to dance CUBAN HIP MOVEMENT.

Next . . . practice moving around the room doing DOUBLE RHYTHM. The call will be "SIDE TOGETHER . . . SIDE TOGETHER . . . etc." Start with the LEFT FOOT and the Left foot will be free for each new UNIT.

COUNT:	1 2	3 4	5 6	7 8
UNIT:	[● ●]	[● ●]	[● ●]	[● ●]
VERBAL:	"SIDE TOGETHER. . .	SIDE TOGETHER. . .	SIDE TOGETHER. . .	SIDE TOGETHER"
FOOT:	L R	L R	L R	L R
HIP:	R L	R L	R L	R L

UNDERARM TURN

HE does a Basic BOX STEP turning gradually LEFT. HE maintains the BOX STEP through EIGHT UNITS (16 beats of music) (2 SETS of 8 counts)

HE: lifts his LEFT hand as he steps BACK on his right foot. (count 7)

SHE: She walks Forward on count 7, under his left hand and continues walking forward in a large CW (clockwise) circle through counts 1 2 3 hold 4 . . . 5 6 7 hold 8.
Both partners are now in position to repeat a basic BOX to close the position.

Practice these first two patterns to RUMBA music and then to a slow CONTEMPORARY sound. This is considered BOX RUMBA and is danced as a basic in most social dance curriculums.

Maintaining the RHYTHM and the STYLE of the dance so far . . . practice moving from CLOSED DANCE POSITION to open TWO HAND POSITION . . . and then into a CRADLE POSITION. From there WALK in a circle, both partners walking FORWARD to form a revolving WHEEL. From there you could go into a PRETZEL POSITION and revolve again. This new concept allows the RUMBA to move easily from standard to contemporary dance floors. The INTERPRETATION will vary with the MUSIC, but the effect will be the same.

Other variations in RUMBA, consist of taking the CHA CHA patterns and changing all of the TRIPLE RHYTHM UNITS to SINGLE RHYTHM. If the tempo is MAMBO, you will be dancing MAMBO. If the tempo is medium or SLOW, you will be dancing OPEN RUMBA (or Mambolero). For TEACHERS and ADVANCED STUDENTS OF THE DANCE:

In the G.S.D.T.A. curriculum, RUMBA is considered to be in the CHA CHA, MAMBO family and when it is danced OPEN STYLE, it "BREAKS ON TWO." (see CHA CHA.) Many of the teachers actually teach BOX RHYTHM starting the SIDE TOGETHER on the TWO BEAT. At present, examinations allow either ONE or TWO for RUMBA but insist on the TWO BEAT for CHA CHA or MAMBO. The more progressive teacher might wish to start teaching the BOX RUMBA to the side on TWO. That will be the coming thing. By starting on the TWO COUNT . . . the dance can move easily from BOX RUMBA into OPEN RUMBA. BOLERO also breaks on TWO in the G.S.D.T.A. curriculum, making the circle complete . . . and continuing the feeling of the TWO BEAT through all of the RUMBA FAMILY.

It would seem that not much space has been allotted to the RUMBA. However, the accent is on CONTEMPORARY SOCIAL DANCE . . . both in BALLROOM DANCING and in NITE CLUB DANCING. The RUMBA has almost become ABSORBED in the other Latin Dances. One can adapt the CHA CHA patterns . . . the NEW YORK HUSTLE positions and do more variations than one could use in a lifetime.

The CONCEPT of this book is to give the reader (STUDENT or TEACHER) the foundation from which to build. If the individual is particularly interested in more specific patterns, each dance has a STEP PATTERN LIST of FORTY or MORE PATTERNS . . . not counting the RHYTHM and STYLE VARIATIONS. Each dance is available in a more detailed form in NOTEBOOK FORM. This is ideal for a TEACHER or ADVANCED STUDENT who is interested in DETAILED STEP PATTERNS.

However, the average dancer, dancing SOCIALLY will have more material from this book than he will ever need.

RECAP . . .

- RUMBA alternates DOUBLE and SINGLE RHYTHM
- The CHARACTERISTIC of the dance is the CUBAN HIP STYLING
- OPEN RUMBA "BREAKS on the TWO BEAT."
- BOX RUMBA starts to the SIDE with DOUBLE RHYTHM.
- The UPPER BODY LIFTS as the CPB follows the MOVING FOOT

WALTZ

Have you ever watched a floor full of waltzers and noticed that even though they were all doing BASICALLY the same patterns, that only one or two couples really "floated" across the floor? Although Waltz is considered one of the easier dances to do, a mastery of the dance requires much more than just patterns.

The basic MOVEMENT of a Waltz is the rise and fall. The first beat of every forward measure is stepped with the heel first, rolling onto the ball of the foot and rising for steps "2" and "3." As you step BACK on the first beat of a measure, the toe hits first and "melts" to the heel. The "2" count is a rise with an even higher rise on "3."

At all times, the back is straight and tall, with the shoulders leaning slightly BACK of center point of balance. One partner balances the other. Assuming an "attitude" does wonders for Waltz. Tell yourself, "I'm the tallest, best looking person on the floor." Put your chin out, head up — and GO!

All of the Basic level patterns can be divided into two categories: A Waltz step (stepping on all three counts), and a Balance step (stepping on "1" and holding the 2-3). The easiest method of remembering patterns and staying on the correct foot is to count your Waltz in "measures." We have a LEFT MEASURE and a RIGHT MEASURE. Waltz is played in 3/4 time (three quarter notes to a measure). If we count in measures, the "verbal" breakdown will be: "Left-2-3 — Right-2-3." This eliminates the possibility of stepping on the wrong foot at the end of a measure.

In Waltz, there are "heavy" measures and "light" measures. You will notice that the patterns are EVEN numbers of measures. Thus, if a new pattern STARTS on the HEAVY measure, it will ensure automatic phrasing.

As is true of most dances, a few steps done well are far more effective than a wide variety done without sufficient knowledge and control to make them comfortable.

Learning to Waltz helps develop a better sense of BALANCE. Each dance helps the overall dance picture by contributing some important motion or control that is not as prevalent in the other dances. This is the reason many dancers work on ALL the dances, even though they confine their dancing pleasure to a selected few.

The patterns written here are for medium tempo, American Waltz. Faster Waltz becomes Viennese and Slower Waltz becomes International Style. Both are popular versions, but the "old standard" medium tempo is still the most danced and most popular.

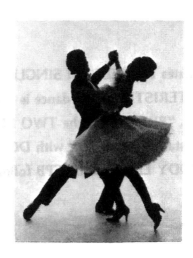

A UNIT = 2 Beats of Music

A UNIT with ONE STRIPE = 3 beats of music
3 Beats of Music = 1 WALTZ MEASURE

WALTZ . . . 3/4 Time . . . Separated in MEASURES instead of UNITS

	1 2 3		4 5 6

Triple Rhythm Measures:

OR

Step Step Step Step Step Step

Single Rhythm Measures:

Step (Tch Hold) Step (Tch Hold)

    All Primary Waltz patterns will be composed of alternating TRIPLES. Secondary patterns include SINGLES . . . (Step Tch) . . . (Hesitation) . . . (Balance). Advanced patterns include Syncopations.

BASIC RULES

    Read the Basic Rules first. These will apply for all the patterns listed unless otherwise specified.

1. All Basic patterns listed are 2 measures (6 beats of music).

2. Man's left foot will start on the heavy measure (Lady's right).

3. The first step listed is a Waltz Box step. This first pattern is done in an actual square so that you can SEE the box. This is only an exercise. Once you start DANCING, the box will take various shapes as it turns Left or Right or proceeds diagonally down line of dance.

4. The FORWARD step for each partner will be BETWEEN the feet of the other partner (directly under the C.P.B. of partner).

5. The Basic Movement   D.U.U.   is Down on count one — 2/3 of the way up on count two — and all the way up on count three. (If you are all the way up on TWO, there will be a tendency to drop on 3 instead of AFTER the 3.)

6. Step HEEL first (flat of the heel) on all FORWARD counts of ONE or FOUR. The footwork "CALL" is "HEEL — TOE — TOE."

7. The movement of UP is the pressing of the ball of the foot into the floor (common usage of "TOE" actually means BALL OF THE FOOT). To be on one's toes would be restrictive. (See terminology.)

8. The "C.P.B." will lean in the direction of the MEASURE foot.
  (Say "Left-2-3 — Right-2-3) "Lean to the Left — Lean to the Right."

9. Remember that the shoulders do not do the leaning. Think into the CENTER (solar plexus). (See Chapter on Movement.)

10. The shoulders will be on a slight diagonal. Pull LEFT Shoulder BACK as you step FORWARD on the LEFT FOOT. Hold that shoulder position through counts 2 and 3. (This is Contra-Body movement.)

		1 2 3	4 5 6

WALTZ MEASURE . . . ▮●●● ▮●●●

		1 2 3	4 5 6	
1.	**LEFT BOX TURN:** Foot:	Fwd Side Tog L R L	Back Side Tog R L R	(Gradually turning Left)
	LADY: Foot:	Back Side Tog R L R	Fwd Side Tog L R L	
2.	**PROGRESSIVE:** Foot:	Fwd Side Tog L R L	Fwd Side Tog R L R	(All Forward) L.O.D.
	LADY: Foot:	Back Side Tog R L R	Back Side Tog L R L	
3.	**RIGHT BOX TURN:** Foot:	Back Side Tog L R L	Fwd Side Tog R L R	(Gradually turning Right)
	LADY: Foot:	Fwd Side Tog R L R	Back Side Tog L R L	
4.	**SINGLE TWINKLE:** Foot:	Fwd Side Tog L R L	Fwd Side Tog R L R	(Close the position on 5-6)
	LADY: Foot:	Back Side Tog R L R	Fwd Side Tog L R L	

(On "together" of first unit . . . BOTH partners face LOD (Conversation Position), and BOTH travel FORWARD on the 2nd Measure.)

5.   Now — Go back to each pattern and replace the 1st Measure with a SINGLE RHYTHM MEASURE . . . Step & Hold or Step Point (leaving out the "side together").

 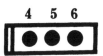

6.   Now — go back and reverse the Order.

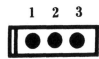 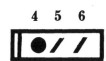

WALTZ MEASURE . . .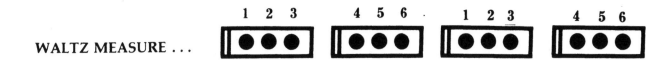

7. **UNDERARM TURN:**

MAN:	Fwd Side Tog	Back Side Tog	Fwd Side Tog	Back Side Tog
(2 Left Box Turns)				
FOOT:	L R L	R L R	L R L	R L R

(gradual CC, Left turn on 1 & 5)

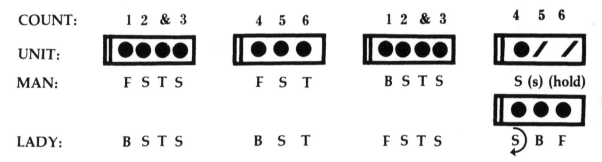

LADY:	Back Side Tog	Fwd Fwd Fwd	Fwd Fwd Fwd	Fwd Side Tog
(6 Walking Steps on #2 and #3)				
FOOT:	R L R	L R L	R L R	L R L
MEASURE:	#1	#2	#3	#4

Man lifts LEFT hand at beginning of 2nd measure and lady walks straight forward into large circle for 2 measures. (Man keeps turning LEFT.)

8. Now it's time for some fun with an EXTENDED DOUBLE (FOUR STEPS to 3 beats).

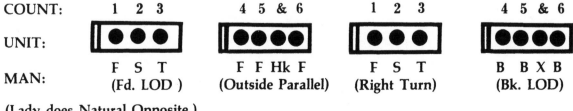

COUNT:	1 2 & 3	4 5 6	1 2 & 3	4 5 6
MAN:	F S T S	F S T	B S T S	S (s) (hold)
LADY:	B S T S	B S T	F S T S	S) B F

(Entire pattern is a gradual turn LEFT. Man starts facing LOD and finishes with his Back to the Center, Fanning the Lady to his RIGHT. Follow this pattern with a LEFT BOX TURN, placing the Lady in front of the man on count ONE.)

It is important when doing an EVEN MEASURE (4 steps or two steps) to REPEAT an EVEN MEASURE to return the man to the DOMINANT POSITION of stepping Forward on the first beat of a HEAVY MEASURE.

9. FORWARD and BACK LOCKS (Reverses the RHYTHM of the above Pattern.)

COUNT:	1 2 3	4 5 & 6	1 2 3	4 5 & 6
MAN:	F S T	F F Hk F	F S T	B B X B
	(Fd. LOD)	(Outside Parallel)	(Right Turn)	(Bk. LOD)

(Lady does Natural Opposite.)

SUGGESTED AMALGAMATIONS:

	# of Measures:
2 LEFT BOX TURNS (Starting LOD/ Ending Diagonal to Right Wall.)	4
2 PROGRESSIVE BOX STEPS turning the LAST measure to the RIGHT.	4
2 RIGHT BOX TURNS (end w/Man facing RIGHT wall.)	4
1 SINGLE TWINKLE (ends w/Man still facing RIGHT wall.)	2
1 Forward Balance and Back Waltz to face LOD.	2
	16

Practice doing the FIRST EIGHT MEASURES.

Then practice the SECOND EIGHT MEASURES.

Make sure you can do each set WELL before putting the two together.

Recap:

- Learn each pattern by itself.
- Repeat each pattern several times.
- Combine TWO patterns.
- Put them all together in SETS of EIGHT MEASURES EACH.
- Compose your own SETS on paper and see how creative you can be.

Check Quiz:

1. How many beats of music in a Waltz Measure?_____

2. Forward steps are danced in which foot position?_____

3. Is the RISE on count TWO as high as count THREE?_____

4. Is WALTZ only danced in SINGLE and TRIPLE RHYTHM MEA-SURES?_____

5. A Basic Rule of Movement is that the weight stays over the UNIT FOOT. Is this also true of a WALTZ MEASURE?_____

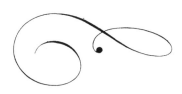

"WEST COAST SWING" ... "GOLDEN STATE SWING"

By whatever name one wishes to call it ... SWING is a dance that is here to stay. The STYLES change ... the MUSIC changes according to the "beat" of the day. But the DANCE is as AMERICAN as apple pie ... and that will go on forever! Many people consider SWING as AMERICA'S ONLY TRUE FOLK DANCE. It was BORN HERE and has grown up in different parts of the country much the same as any child. People from different parts of the country have varying vocabularies ... accents ... life styles ... etc. It is easy to understand then, why different parts of the country produce different STYLES of SWING DANCERS. But a SWING DANCER is a SWING DANCER ... no matter what the style. The most fascinating part of SWING DANC-ING is the individuality of the dancer.

In school, one teacher teaches many children how to write ... Still NO TWO SIGNATURES ARE THE SAME. The same dance teacher teaches many people to dance ... still no two dancers are exactly the same. PATTERNS are taught to learn to move with ease in all direc-tions. STYLING comes from knowing the patterns so well that the mind no longer needs to think about the pattern. STYLINGS are flexible. While the BASIC FORM of the dance should conform to some degree ... the STYLE one chooses should be as individual as the clothes one chooses to wear. We all know individuals who dress in poor taste ... or who dress in excellent taste. (We seldom notice the ones in between ... Right?) The same is true of the dance. "Try on" different styles that you admire in other people ... until you find the comfortable one that FITS YOU. Like so many things in life ... we get from dancing exactly what we put into it.

Patterns in dance are taught to give someone a foundation on which to build. SWING offers such a variety of RHYTHM and STYLE VARIATIONS that eventually each dancer develops his own unique interpretation. The only problem that exists in SWING is when someone decides that there is only ONE WAY to dance it. There is never only ONE WAY to do anything ... or time would stand still and none of us would grow. All dance forms are in a constant stage of growth. SWING is no exception.

The patterns listed here are from the GOLDEN STATE DANCE TEACHERS CUR-RICULUM. The G.S.D.T.A. has been noted through the years for having one of the most com-prehensive and UP-TO-DATE curriculums available. The most important aspect for a student is: how EASILY CAN I LEARN IT? ... how QUICKLY can I learn it? ... and, how can I pass up the stage of looking like a beginner?

The answers are all in the following curriculum. Usually, every beginner SWING dancer gets stuck in a basic pattern, starting in closed position, and seems to have difficulty going from there. This curriculum STARTS in OPEN POSITION for Grade I and teaches you how to start in CLOSED POSITION in Grade II. (Teachers of Dance, please note: This method allows the student to learn the first 4 or 5 patterns in the FIRST LESSON.)

There are a few BASIC RULES for learning QUICKLY and EASILY. USE THE RULES. Later on you can experiment and add RHYTHM VARIATIONS and STYLE VARIA-TIONS. Variations are unlimited ... but sticking to the BASICS FIRST will reward you with a greater understanding and execution of the dance.

1. SHE ... will always start with the RIGHT FOOT ... HE ... with the LEFT.

2. Each pattern will start on a DOWN BEAT. (counts ONE or THREE of a measure.)

3. SHE ... will walk FORWARD FORWARD on the first TWO BEATS of EVERY PATTERN.

4. SHE ... will step THREE TIMES for counts 3&4 in varying foot positions ... but MOST of the time she can think "Right behind the Left" for her RIGHT TRIPLE.

5. SHE ... will STEP THREE TIMES in 3rd foot position, (Left foot behind the Right) for the LAST UNIT of every pattern. (Counts 5&6 in a 6 beat pattern ... or counts 7&8 in an 8 beat pattern.) This is the "ANCHOR."

6. SHE ... will have a RHYTHM PATTERN (to start) of SIX BEATS of music: DOU-BLE ... (Walk Walk) ... a RIGHT TRIPLE (R behind the L) and a LEFT TRIPLE ("Anchor" L behind the R.)

113

7. HE . . . will practice his two TRIPLES (counts 3&4 . . . and 5&6) by standing in 3rd foot position (Left foot in front of the Right) and doing the following VERBAL PATTERN: "STEP TOGETHER FORWARD and ANCHOR IN PLACE."
   L   R   L   and   R   L   R

8. HE . . . will vary his FIRST UNIT according to the location of his partner:

   a. If SHE is BEHIND HIM (or in closed position) his FIRST STEP on count ONE will be FORWARD.

   b. If SHE is in FRONT of him (facing him) his FIRST STEP on count ONE of the pattern will be BACK.

   Later style variations allow several choices of direction for the man but the above will get him moving FASTER and SOONER. . . .
   (The #8. Rule is easy to remember if you think of it this way: No matter where SHE is . . . HE is running away. Ha!)

9. The only count left for the MAN is count TWO. Count TWO is determined by the direction of the PATTERN. COUNT TWO will be the "variable."

Think of the patterns as being danced in a SLOT. (This makes for easy maneuvering on a tight floor.) The MAN is the center of the SLOT. SHE travels up and down the SLOT as if she were on roller skates. HER CPB is sent back and forth as if on a giant RUBBER BAND. The LEVERAGE (resistance) consists of changing her direction at given points in the pattern. This INTERACTION between the two bodies produces BODY FLIGHT.

• LEARN the FIRST FOUR PATTERNS and then put them together as an amalgamation:

#1. UNDERARM TURN:

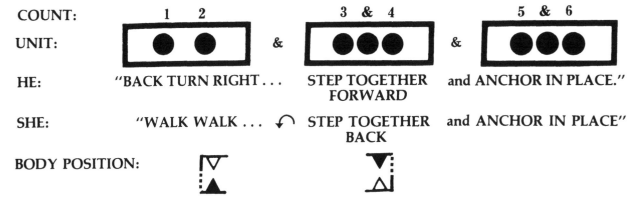

(Man lifts his LEFT hand on count TWO. She TURNS LEFT on the "and" count between 2 and 3) She goes under her OWN Right hand.

* #2. LEFT SIDE PASS: (MAN'S LEFT HAND STAYS LOW ON THE PASS.)

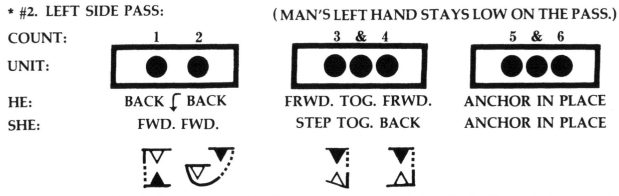

* NOTE: In SWING the use of FWD. TOG FWD. . . . and BK TOG BK on the TRIPLES, refers to OPEN and CLOSED THIRD FOOT POSITION instead of 4th and 1st.

#3. TURNING BASIC:

COUNT:	1 2	3 & 4	5 & 6
UNIT:	● ●	● ● ●	● ● ●

HE: "BACK TURN RT.   BK. PLACE FWD.   and ANCHOR IN PLACE"

(He catches the girl with his RIGHT HAND on count THREE.)

SHE: "FWD. FWD.   BK TOG FWD.   BK TOG BACK"

(She catches his RIGHT ARM with her LEFT HAND on count THREE.)

#4. SLINGSHOT THROWOUT:

COUNT:	1 2	3 & 4	5 & 6
HE:	"FWD. BACK	FWD. TOG FWD.	ANCHOR IN PLACE"
SHE:	"FWD. FWD.	BK TOG BACK	ANCHOR IN PLACE"

AMALGAMATIONS are more fun when they phrase to the music. SWING MUSIC phrases to FOUR counts of EIGHT. (8 Measures of four beats each.) Here's an easy way to make these patterns PHRASE and also learn how to use a LINK. Each ROW is 4 UNITS (8 Beats of music.)

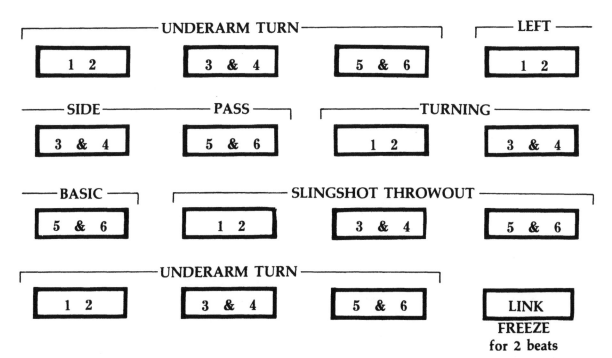

     ...and start over. Listen to any "steady beat" music. Wait for the start of a new PHRASE. You will begin to recognize the phrasing the same as you hear someone end a sentence. There is a BREATH ... or PAUSE that gets ready to start again.

#5. FREEZE . . . A Basic Freeze is just STANDING STILL for two beats of music. In the above amalgamation this ONE UNIT FREEZE has been used as a LINK to make the amalgamation fit the PHRASING OF THE MUSIC. To add a STOP TIME LINK to any pattern, just FREEZE THE POSITION for two beats of music. The man can lead this from an underarm turn by completing the pattern . . . THEN . . . Place the hand FIRMLY DOWN and in a frozen position. The girl will either STOP entirely for the two beats of music or may do a FIRST BREAK ENDING (delayed DOUBLE) waiting for him to start again.

#6. UNDERARM CATCH . . . (an alternative to the TURNING BASIC)

The UNDERARM CATCH is the same as an UNDERARM TURN EXCEPT that the man catches her around the waist on count THREE and keeps her in CLOSED POSITION through count SIX. (Follow with a SLINGSHOT THROWOUT.)

#7. PUSH BREAK (Formerly Sugarpush) 2 hand lead starts in OPEN POSITION.

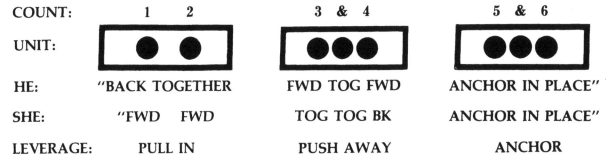

COUNT:	1 2	3 & 4	5 & 6
HE:	"BACK TOGETHER	FWD TOG FWD	ANCHOR IN PLACE"
SHE:	"FWD FWD	TOG TOG BK	ANCHOR IN PLACE"
LEVERAGE:	PULL IN	PUSH AWAY	ANCHOR

(The resistance starts on count TWO is strongest on count THREE and changes the girl's direction on count FOUR.) The PUSHBREAK seems very simple in its STEP PATTERN. However, it is the LEVERAGE . . . the RESISTANCE that makes the pattern. There should be no excessive PUSHING or PULLING in the arms but in the BODY. The arms should remain FIRM but FLEXIBLE.

The ACTION and REACTION of this pattern is the gentle pressure of the Hands bringing the girl TOWARD the man on the FIRST UNIT (count ONE TWO) . . . followed by the pressure FORWARD on the SECOND UNIT (count 3 & 4) SHE is the REACTION: "Pull yourself forward and Push away and Anchor."

* #8. TWO UNIT PREPARATORY (start in closed position)
Partners hinged at HIS RIGHT HIP and HER LEFT HIP.
HIS LEFT HAND, palm up . . . at waist level.
HER RIGHT HAND placed in his Left Hand.
HIS RIGHT HAND cradles her back.
HER LEFT HAND gently holds his Right Arm.

COUNT:	1 2		3 & 4
HE:	Fwd (tch)		Anchor In Place
SHE:	Fwd (tch)	&	BK TOG BK

NOTE: There are only FOUR BEATS. This is just a STARTER STEP. Follow with a Slingshot Throwout. Rearrange your Amalgamation to suit.

---

*TEACHERS: Students should be dancing steps 1 thru 7 with ease, before being introduced to the TWO UNIT PREPARATORY. A VERBAL CALL for this pattern might be "GET READY . . . GET SET" and "GO" on count one of the THROWOUT.

There are numerous "TUCK-INS." Following the basic rules described earlier, the only change of pattern is in the LEAD for the man . . . and in the 1st TRIPLE for the girl. For ANY "TUCK-IN" from closed position . . . open position . . . one hand lead . . . two hand lead . . . the TUCK itself is the same.: (it is on THREE and FOUR)

COUNT:	1	2	3 & 4	5 and 6
HER CPB:	FWD	FWD	"Turn Left Turn Right"	& Anchor in place.
HER FOOT POSITIONS:	4th	4th	4th 1st 4th	3rd

SHE can practice a TUCK IN by doing the FOOT PLACEMENT without the turn:

COUNT:	1 2	3 & 4	5 & 6
VERBAL:	FWD FWD	FWD TOG FWD	ANCHOR IN PLACE

THEN practice the . . . . . . FWD TOG FWD turning LEFT on 3 and RIGHT on 4.

Although there are many THREE UNIT PATTERNS (6 beats) it is also important to be aware of the FOUR UNIT RHYTHM PATTERN (WHIP RHYTHM) (8 beats)

#1. WHIP RELEASE:

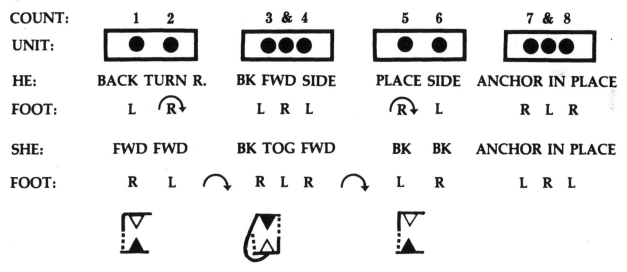

COUNT:	1 2	3 & 4	5 6	7 & 8
HE:	BACK TURN R.	BK FWD SIDE	PLACE SIDE	ANCHOR IN PLACE
FOOT:	L R↴	L R L	R↴ L	R L R
SHE:	FWD FWD	BK TOG FWD	BK BK	ANCHOR IN PLACE
FOOT:	R L	R L R	L R	L R L

HE catches girl on count THREE and releases her as he turns RIGHT on count FOUR.

⤶ =Left or CCW turn

⤷ =Right or clockwise turn

117

#2. CLOSED WHIP: (formerly called a Lindy Turn) (a WHIP with NO RELEASE)

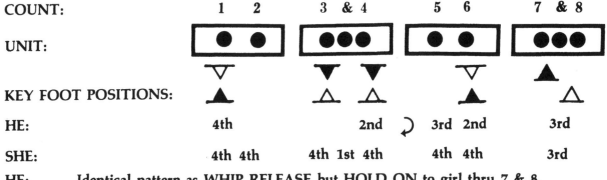

COUNT:	1 2	3 & 4	5 6	7 & 8
HE:	4th	2nd	3rd 2nd	3rd
SHE:	4th 4th	4th 1st 4th	4th 4th	3rd

HE: Identical pattern as WHIP RELEASE but HOLD ON to girl thru 7 & 8.

SHE: Same as WHIP for the first TWO UNITS . . . Do a BACK FORWARD for counts 5-6 and

anchor   **BACK TOGETHER BACK**   for 7 & 8.

#3. WHIP WITH HAND CHANGE:

Standard Whip . . . but man changes hands behind the girl's back on count FOUR. Keep the man's LEFT hand in close to the body on counts TWO and THREE so that there will be no resistance for the FOUR. Change hands back to original on counts 7 & 8. (or can follow with a RIGHT HAND WHIP.)

#4. RIGHT HAND WHIP:

Man's part is IDENTICAL to a regular WHIP except that he leads with his RIGHT HAND.

SHE, however, must turn LEFT instead of RIGHT on the "and" between 2 & 3 in order to do a complete ½ turn to complete her "BACK TOGETHER FORWARD" on counts 3 & 4. By locking her feet in 4th foot position for counts 5 & 6 she will roll out in a 4th foot position pivot to end with an ANCHOR.

WEST COAST SWING being one of the dances that the GSDTA has been noted for . . . we have some 200 or more patterns and variations in this dance alone . . . and that would be another book in itself. (and will be available in booklet form for the 1979 semester.)

However, the material offered here is a good start toward becoming an accomplished SWING DANCER. The REPRINT SHEETS that follow will give you ideas on additional patterns and RHYTHM VARIATIONS. Don't just READ THEM . . . DANCE THEM!

FOR STARTERS:

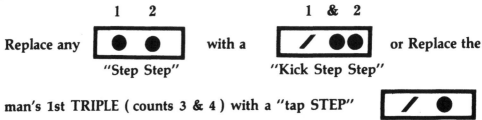

Replace any   "Step Step"   with a   "Kick Step Step"   or Replace the

man's 1st TRIPLE (counts 3 & 4) with a "tap STEP"

A SUGARPUSH is a THREE UNIT PATTERN. A "DOUBLE SUGARPUSH" is SIX UNITS. An easy version of a DOUBLE SUGARPUSH is to insert a THIRD BREAK ENDING for UNITS number THREE and FOUR:

1 2	3 4	& 5 & 6 &	1 & 2	3 4	5 & 6
● ●	╱ ●	◐╱◐╱◐	╱● ●	╱ ●	● ● ●

                                           Stp.(K)St.(K)Stp.   (K)Stp.Stp.

DIR. of KICKS: (F)   (B)   (F)

RESISTANCE:

Back   Fwd.   (B) (F)   (B) F   (F) F   "Anchor"

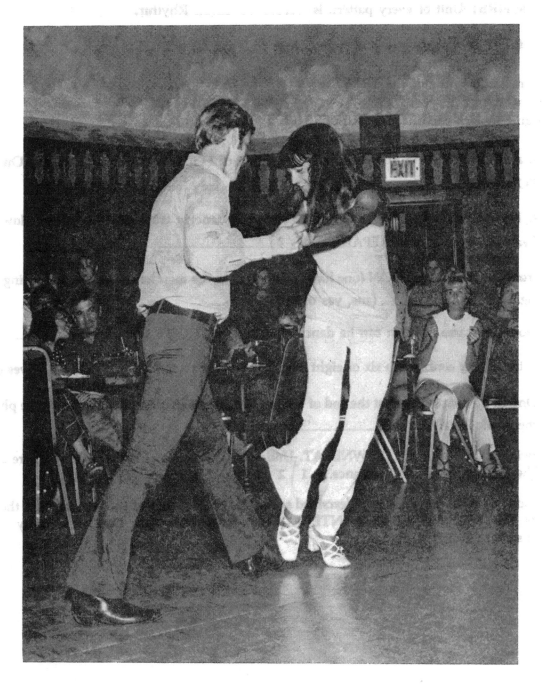

QUIZ:

1. West Coast Swing is primarily a SLOT dance. On counts ONE and TWO of the lady's part, she steps: FORWARD FORWARD or BACK FORWARD?
   _____ _____.

2. Basic Patterns contain how many UNITS? _____

3. The ANCHOR UNIT is the 1st or last UNIT of every pattern? _____

4. The FIRST Unit of every pattern is _____ Rhythm.

5. A WHIP is composed of how many Units? _____

6. Can I replace one of the TRIPLES with a "tap STEP"? _____

7. Can I replace one of the DOUBLES with a "tap STEP"? _____

8. In a SUGARPUSH (a PUSH BREAK) the count of FOUR is the strongest move. On count FOUR the man moves _____ and the lady moves _____.

9. A TWO UNIT PREPARATORY is used to start dancing from closed position. How many beats of music in the PREPARATORY? _____

10. From an OPEN POSITION (one hand contact) does the man have a choice of turning left or right? _____ (ans. yes or no)

11. From that same position can he dance a pattern WITHOUT turning? _____

12. Is the dancer confined to six or eight beat patterns in Swing? _____ (yes or no)

13. One UNIT that is added at the end of a series of patterns in order to make the dance phrase to the music is called a _____.

14. Swing is danced on the DOWNBEAT. Underline the counts of the measure that are considered the DOWNBEATS in the dance.: 1   2   3   4 .

15. Body Flight in Swing has been described as the INTERACTION of the two bodies of the dancers. Is this BODY FLIGHT or INTERACTION something that can be seen by an ob-observer? _____.

Golden State Dance Teachers Association

Prepared for SAN DIEGO BICENTENNIAL SWING DANCE
FESTIVAL, ••• SKIPPY BLAIR ••• May 29, 1976 •••

SUGAR PUSH VARIATION

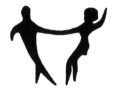

HIS PATTERN:

COUNT:	1	2		3	4		&	5	6
UNIT:	●	●		/	●		●/	/	
FOOT:	L	R		(L)	L		R		
DIRECTION:	B	T		(F)	F		F		
VERBAL:	"Pull and			(Point) Step			Step point hold"		

HER PATTERN:

COUNT:	1	2		3	4		&	5	6
UNIT:	●	●		/	●		●/	/	
FOOT:	R	L		(R)	R		L	(R)	
DIRECTION:	F	F		(F)	B		X	(B)	
VERBAL:	"Walk Walk			Kick Step Back			Cross Point & hold."		

The MOVEMENT UNIT for BOTH PARTNERS is the same:

1st UNIT . . . BOTH PARTNERS "pull back" (leverage from body movement)
2nd UNIT . . . BOTH PARTNERS "push away"
3rd UNIT . . . NEUTRAL . . . the "ANCHOR UNIT."

Having shown the COMPLETE PATTERN above, the following UNITS can be substituted for counts 5&6 . . . (or ANY triple in ANY pattern)

COUNT:	& 5 & 6 &		& 5 & 6 &		5 6 &
	●/●/●	OR	●●●●●	OR	/ /●
	Syncopated TRIPLE:		EXTENDED TRIPLE:		Sync. DELAYED SINGLE:

VERBAL: "Step KICK Step KICK Step" (5 little steps)   "KICK Swivel Step"

We can also replace TWO UNITS of a pattern by changing the rhythm entirely. In an UNDERARM TURN. The Lady can do:

COUNT:	1	2		& 3 & 4		& 5 & 6
	●	●		●●●●		●●●●
VERBAL:	"WALK WALK"			"Side Tog. Side Tog."		"Side Tog. Side Tog."

. . .OR . . . EITHER partner can replace the FIRST UNIT of any pattern with a DELAYED DOUBLE. That is called a FIRST BREAK ENDING . . . or a HITCH KICK:

COUNT:	1 & 2
	/●●

VERBAL: "KICK Step Step"

> Note: The SYNCOPATED TRIPLE above, followed by a DELAYED DOUBLE . . . becomes a THIRD BREAK ENDING.

Golden State Dance Teachers Association

SWING AND/OR CALIFORNIA SHUFFLE

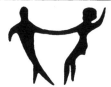

REPRINT

• San Diego Swing Convention . . . May 1978, SAN DIEGO SWING CLUB.
• WORKSHOP NOTES for presentation by SKIPPY BLAIR.

There is a CONTEMPORARY STYLE of SYNCOPATED SWING that is fast gaining favor with the younger generation. It is very UP and very SOPHISTICATED . . . and, I might add . . . very much FUN. The notes printed below are very easy to read if you take the time to look at the DOTS. Each DOT is a STEP . . . a weight change. Each SLASH is a (KICK) or a (POINT) but (NO WEIGHT CHANGE). It is as simple as that. The UNIVERSAL UNIT SYSTEM is a method of breaking down ANY DANCE MATERIAL in EASY TO READ form. The COUNT is the ACTUAL BEATS OF MUSIC that it takes to complete the pattern.

(For those already familiar with the system, the patterns listed below are merely extensions of an UNDERARM TURN, SUGARPUSH and a LEFT TUCK. These three SIX BEAT PATTERNS have been extended to become EIGHT BEAT PATTERNS.)

COUNT:	1 2	3 & 4	& 5 & 6 &	7 & 8 &
UNIT:	●●	●●●	●/●/●	/●/●
Name of Unit:	DOUBLE	TRIPLE	SYNCOPATED TRIPLE	SYNCOPATED DOUBLE
HE STEPS: (point)	L R	L R L	R L R (L) (R)	L R (L) (R)
SHE STEPS: (point)	R L	R L R	L R L (R) (L)	R L (R) (L)

The SAME COUNT and the SAME VERBAL PATTERN for WEIGHT CHANGES applies to several variations of the same syncopation. The VERBAL PATTERN or "CALL" could be:

1 2   3 & 4   5   6   7   8
*"STEP STEP and STEP THREE TIMES . . . STEP POINT STEP POINT STEP POINT STEP POINT STEP."

The KEY to doing the syncopation correctly is to make sure that you get in that last STEP. There are FOUR "POINTS," but FIVE "STEPS" in the syncopation . . . leaving the man's LEFT FOOT free to start again . . . and the lady's RIGHT FOOT FREE to start again.

This same syncopation can be done by either the man OR the lady in any of the WHIP RHYTHM PATTERNS (or can be done by BOTH at the same time). To use it in the WHIP merely substitute the last two units . . . (counts 5 6, 7 & 8) with the above syncopation.

*Some of the newer Dancers will recognize the above Patterns as CALIFORNIA SHUFFLE. The CALIFORNIA SHUFFLE is just a series of "STEP (point) STEP (point) etc." It can be danced ALONE . . . or with a partner. In PARTNER DANCING, it can be as simple as doing two WALKING STEPS, then the SHUFFLE for two or three UNITS . . . and repeat. It can also be done as an extension of WEST COAST SWING as explained above.

INTERESTING NOTE . . . At a recent DISCO DEMONSTRATION at J. C. Penneys, one of the managers asked if I could do CALIFORNIA SWING. I said that I could and also added that the CALIFORNIA SHUFFLE is COMPATIBLE with California Swing. Twenty minutes later, we did a DEMONSTRATION. John danced SWING and I danced SHUFFLE to his beat. It brought the house down . . . and we're invited BACK!! (August, 1978)

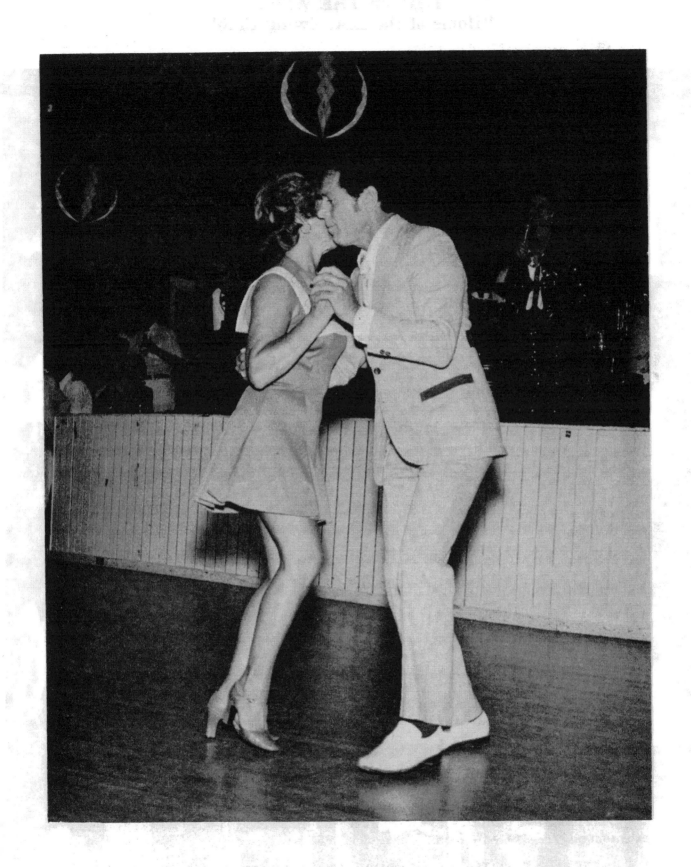

Bart and Natalie "Balboa"
(but it could be California Shuffle)

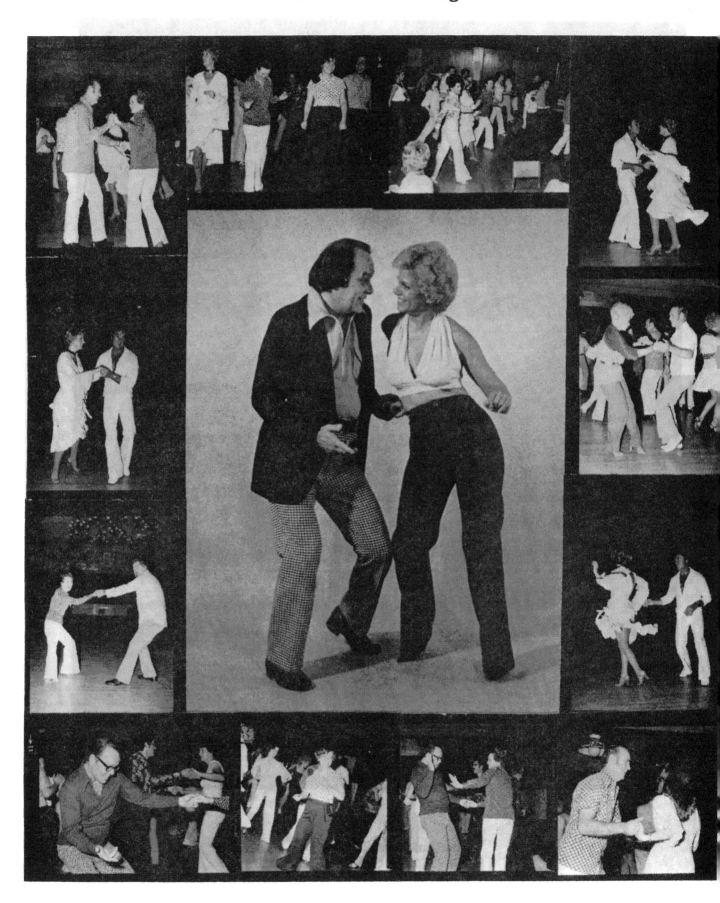

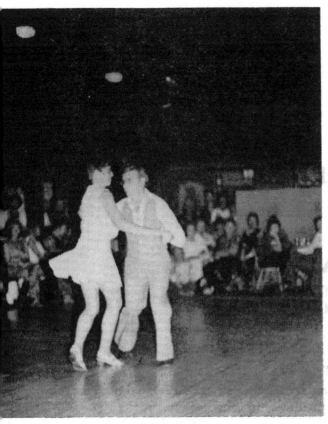

**L.A.S.D.C. Pres.
Tom Boots & Bev**

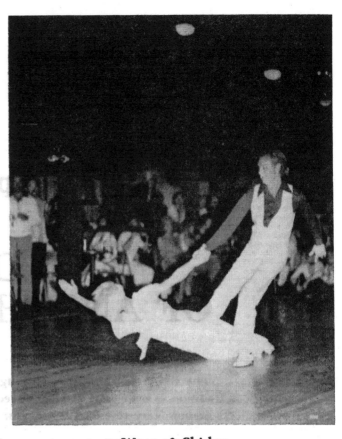

**Wayne & Shirley
"Torpedo"**

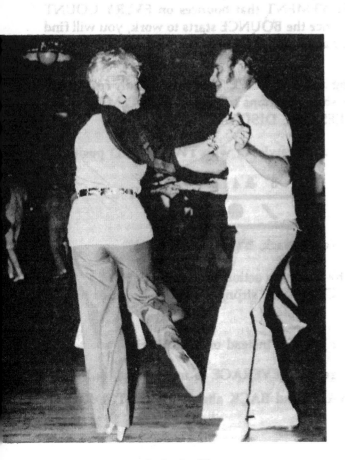

"Kick Swivel"

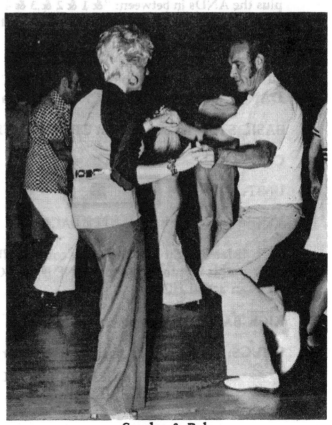

**Sandee & Bob
"Shuffle"**

Chapter IX

FAD DANCES
OF ANOTHER ERA . . .

The CHARLESTON . . . although a FAD DANCE of its day . . . has become an American tradition. It is a classic and can be recognized by almost any age individual whether they are dancers or not. Very few dances can come up to that kind of notoriety.

In its BASIC FORM, the dance could be considered as being composed of all SINGLE RHYTHM: "Step touch and Step touch . . . or . . . Step Kick and Step Kick." However, to dance it properly, one must develop the BOUNCING MOVEMENT that bounces on EVERY COUNT plus the ANDs in between: "& 1 & 2 & 3 & 4 etc. Once the BOUNCE starts to work, you will find that the ACTUAL RHYTHM PATTERN of the Charleston is a DELAYED SINGLE: . . ."(touch) STEP and (touch) STEP"

The CHARLESTON is noted for being a FUN DANCE. One could hardly feel dejected and Dance the Charleston. Many of the Charleston variations surface in CONTEMPORARY DANCE. (evident in the ROCK and now in FREESTYLE DISCO.)

BASIC STEP: (can be done in OPEN POSITION . . . freestyle or with TWO HAND position.)

COUNT:	& 1 & 2 &	3 & 4 &
UNIT:	/ ●	/ ●
VERBAL:	"Touch Fwd, STEP BACK. . .	Touch Back, STEP FORWARD"

(Man's Right foot is free for count ONE. The bouncing action allows him to HOP on his Left foot on count ONE if the BOUNCE becomes strong enough to become an actual HOP.)

KICK BASIC: (Same Pattern can be danced doing a KICK instead of a TOUCH.)

CHUGS: (TWO HAND position is necessary to get the LEVERAGE to move Frwd. & Back.)

(Both feet TOGETHER jump FORWARD and BACK alternating LEFT & RIGHT PARALLEL.

126

The CALL for the man:

"To the RIGHT and back . . . To the LEFT and back. . .
To the RIGHT and to the RIGHT again." (8 counts)

then: "To the LEFT and back . . . to the RIGHT and back. . .
To the LEFT and to the LEFT AGAIN." (8 counts)

The CHARLESTON movement was the forerunner to the BALBOA that was yet to come. The little BOUNCE that is the CHARACTERISTIC of the dance becomes more subtle with practice . . . WALKS . . . HEEL TOE traveling steps . . . all of the interesting little "Show Off" patterns have resurfaced in the late 70s DISCO SCENE.

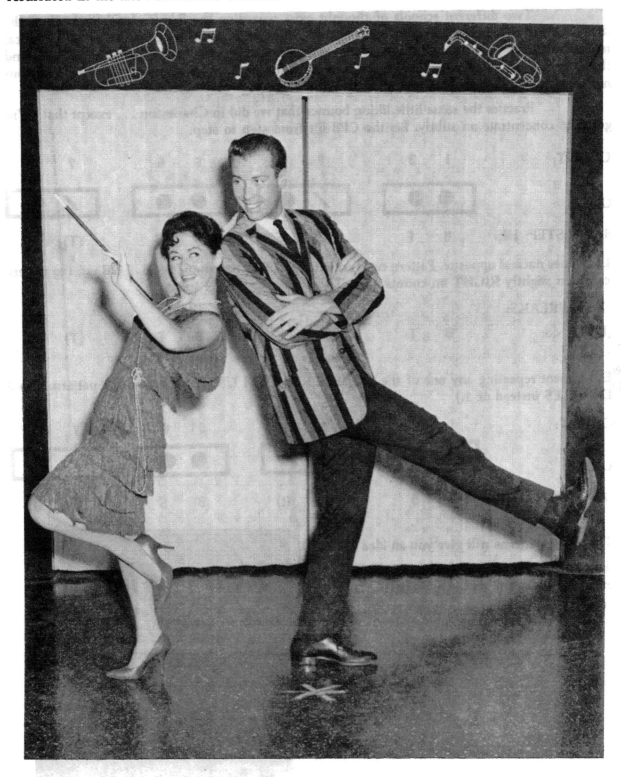

Charleston (1961)   "Little Andy" & John

BALBOA

Balboa is purely a California product . . . started at the Balboa Pavilion during the war years . . . it is still a popular dance with the dancers of the late 30s and the forties. Balboa too has become a classic in the true sense of the word. It has withstood the test of time and a curriculum has developed to the point where it is being taught in social dance classes in the colleges as well as in Studios.

Balboa is really considered a part of SWING. (the shag from St. Louis) Many dancers mix the two dances and they are very compatible. Below are a few basic patterns to give you an idea of the ''feeling'' of the dance.

Two different schools of thought exist regarding the BASIC MOVEMENT of the dance. One says there is NO vertical movement . . . the other says there is a CONSTANT vertical movement. Take your choice. I maintain that movement is necessary to get the dance going . . . and that later, one can remove the EXCESS movement by toning it down to a point where it is FELT but not seen!

Practice the same little lilting bounce that we did in Charleston . . . except that we're going to concentrate on subtly. Let the CPB lilt from step to step.

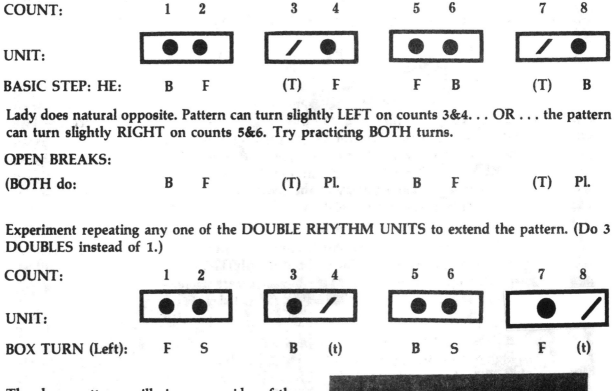

COUNT:	1	2		3	4		5	6		7	8
UNIT:											
BASIC STEP: HE:	B	F		(T)	F		F	B		(T)	B

Lady does natural opposite. Pattern can turn slightly LEFT on counts 3&4 . . . OR . . . the pattern can turn slightly RIGHT on counts 5&6. Try practicing BOTH turns.

OPEN BREAKS:

(BOTH do:	B	F		(T)	Pl.		B	F		(T)	Pl.

Experiment repeating any one of the DOUBLE RHYTHM UNITS to extend the pattern. (Do 3 DOUBLES instead of 1.)

COUNT:	1	2		3	4		5	6		7	8
UNIT:											
BOX TURN (Left):	F	S		B	(t)		B	S		F	(t)

The above patterns will give you an idea of the dance. For more detailed descriptions and extensive variety of patterns, contact
  G.S.D.T.A. Publishers .

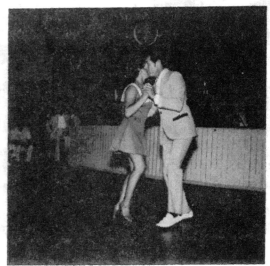

TWIST . . . from "SO YOU WANT TO LEARN TO DANCE ?" ©1963

by Skippy Blair

(with COMMENTS from 1978)

THE TWIST . . . Shades of Chubby Checker!! At this writing, AUGUST 1978, I am including the entire Chapter on TWIST from the 1963 Text book, "SO YOU WANT TO LEARN TO DANCE?" BODY LANGUAGE, currently popular uses MANY of the moves in this Dance. The Patterns also teach a great deal about SWIVELS that are not covered elsewhere. To think CONTEMPORARY . . . just change the KNEE SWING to a HIP SWING. Swinging the knees back and forth made a TWISTING MOTION. The NEW LOOK of BODY LANGUAGE uses HIPS swinging LEFT and RIGHT. (NO Twist.)

Here is the Text . . . Just as it was written in 1962 . . .

All dances, no matter HOW simple, are more interesting, and far more FUN, after you acquire a basic knowledge of technique. EVEN the "TWIST." Like every other dance, the Twist has it's share of devotees. As is the case with ALL new dances, some dancers looked ridiculous, and some actually indecent. However, think of the average dance you've attended lately and ask yourself, "How many REALLY GOOD dancers WERE there?" Narrowing down the field to those who dance WELL, will give you a better picture of the dance, and you will find that ALL dance (including Twist) has a basic form and foundation.

Charleston, once considered quite improper, is now looked upon as "Classic." The Twist as a separate dance, may not last forever, but the MOTION and VARIATIONS will have contributed materially to the other dances. Many Twist dancers can now do SWIVELS in Cha Cha and Swing that they never thought possible before "Twist days."

The RHYTHM PATTERN of Twist is quite different from anything that has come before it. There are FOUR BEATS to the MEASURE, which is certainly not different. The DIFFERENT quality about Twist is that ALL FOUR beats are taken on ONE foot. We refer to a LEFT MEASURE (4 beats) and a RIGHT MEASURE, (4 beats). It is the KNEES that keep the actual COUNT by swinging left and right.

Remember that the basic motion is a TWIST and NOT a WIGGLE!! A simple exercise to show you how easy it can be is this:

*Put the heels together (1st foot position) — Now lift the heels off the floor and bend the knees. Swing the knees to the left and then right — repeat. Easy, isn't it?

1978 Comment . . . The MOVEMENT described here for TWIST is currently being done as a BASIC MOVEMENT for HAND JIVE. (see Contemporary Solo Dancing.)

TWIST (1962)

1. TWIST BASIC

2. REVERSE BASIC

3. ARM STYLINGS

   a. Pendulum

   b. Hinge

4. KNEE LIFT

5. KNEE LIFT CIRCLE

   a. Left

   b. Right

6. CIRCLE SWIVEL

   a. Traveling Left or Right

   b. Spotted Left or Right

7. SIDE BASIC (Two Feet)

8. SIDE BASIC (One Foot)

   a. With simple TOE HEEL action

   b. With KICK forward and back

9. DOUBLE TIME

10. SHIFT

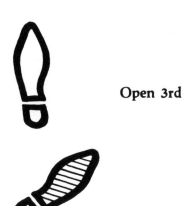 Open 3rd

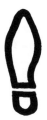 

2nd Foot Position

TWIST BASIC (Open 3rd foot position) starts on LEFT foot

Weight is on:		Left Foot				Right Foot		
COUNT:	1	2	3	4	5	6	7	8
Knees swing:	L	R	L	R	L	R	L	R

REVERSE BASIC: starts on RIGHT foot and knees swing R L

Weight is on:		Right Foot				Left Foot		
COUNT:	1	2	3	4	5	6	7	8
Knees Swing:	R	L	R	L	R	L	R	L

Note that the Man could do a BASIC while girl does a REVERSE BASIC and they would "mesh."

ARM STYLINGS — There are two main arm stylings that are really MORE than just styling. They actaully DO the work for you!

     1. PENDULUM SWING: Let the hands go "heavy." Swing the left arm forward as the right goes back. This "free swing" twists the midriff to set the dance in motion. Put the hands together with the knee motion now and you will have the following:

               LEFT hand swings FORWARD as knees swing LEFT.
               RIGHT hand swings FORWARD as knees go RIGHT.

     2. HINGE: Keep the upper arms firm and swing the forearm left and right to a steady count. This is OPPOSITE arm direction to knee direction. This counter-balances the motion. Hands swing RIGHT as knees go LEFT.

KNEE LIFT - (Open 3rd foot position)

Do first measure (four beats) of Twist Basic — Left Foot.

Second measure — Wt on right foot — Left foot points DOWN on DOWNBEAT (1 & 3) and pulls knee UP on UPBEAT (2 & 4)

COUNT:	1	2	3	4	1	2	3	4
VERBAL:	"Left	2	3	4 —	point	pull	point	pull"

KNEE LIFT CIRCLE

By keeping the weight centered on the RIGHT foot, you can circle Left or circle Right merely by exerting EXTRA FORCE on the UP motion to turn RIGHT — or the DOWN motion to turn LEFT.

```
COUNT:  1    2    3    4    5    6    7    8
Verbal: "point-PULL-pnt-PULL-pnt-PULL-pnt-PULL" (turns right)
Arms:   r    L    r    L    r    L    r    L

OR — "POINT-pull-POINT-pull-POINT-pull-POINT-pull" (turns left)
        R    l    R    l    R    l    R    l
```

This pattern becomes a study in the force of motion. Strangely enough, the motion learned in Twist has led many a dancer into swivels in Cha Cha and Swing that they never thought would be possible!

CIRCLE SWIVEL

Put RIGHT foot in front of left — Now "freeze" the position, and, moving from the HIP (not with the feet), travel LEFT:

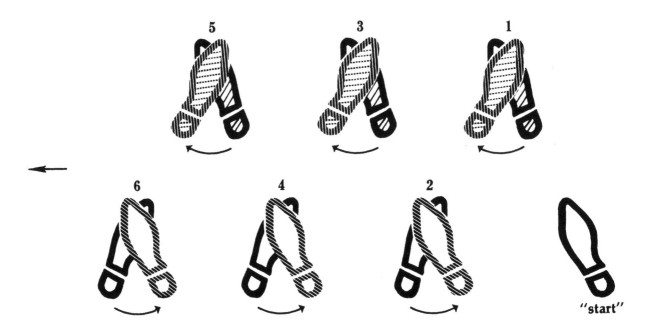

VERBAL: "RIGHT LEFT RIGHT LEFT" etc. changing feet on every count.

You can SPOT the turn by keeping the LEFT FOOT in PLACE and letting the right foot do a "Cross-Swivel" repeat in circle — eight counts.

Traveling or spotted swivels can be done to the RIGHT by putting the LEFT foot FORWARD and reversing the above procedure.

SIDE BASIC (Two Feet)

Verbal:	Toe Heel Toe Heel				Heel Toe Heel Toe				
Direction:	L	L	L	L	R	R	R	R	Repeat
COUNT:	1	2	3	4	5	6	7	8	

Weight shifts from the toes to the heels to move left. Note that the weight is in the HEELS on the 4th count and changes direction, but stays on the heels for the count of "1." The next set finds the change on the toes.

Floor pattern for two feet would make too many footprints superimposed on each other. Imagine then, the right foot directly next to the left — same direction, same weight change:

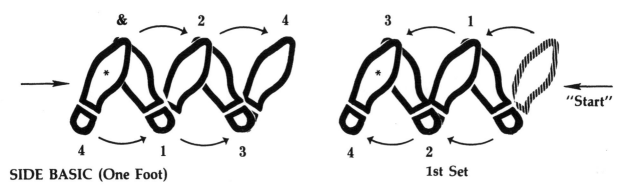

1st Set

SIDE BASIC (One Foot)

Verbal: Same as above
Direction: Same
COUNT: Same

The simple pattern detailed above, can now become quite intricate by a few fairly simple maneuvers. First, do the first set (measure) on the left foot traveling LEFT — shift to RIGHT FOOT to travel RIGHT.

COUNT:	1	2	3	4	&	5	6	7	8	&	
Swivel:					*					*	*No weight change.
Weight:	L	L	L	L	L	R	R	R	R	R	
Toe-Heel:	T	H	T	H	T	H	T	H	T	H	

Note: Free foot rides along in the same direction as the working foot.
1st Variation: touch free foot to floor using same verbal as floor pattern: toe heel toe heel etc.

2nd Variation: Incorporate a "kick" in place of the toe or heel.
"Toe" will become a kick BACK
"Heel" will become a kick FORWARD
Working foot remains the same. Kick comes from the knee down and is merely an extension of the "toe" "Heel" action.

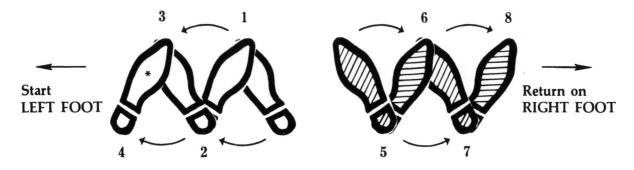

Start
LEFT FOOT

Return on
RIGHT FOOT

DOUBLE TIME (w/circular arm motion)

Done in Basic or Side Basic position, the arms swing in a circular motion from the elbow. The KNEES swing LEFT on EVERY count instead of every OTHER count.

VERBAL:	1	2	3	4	5	6	7	8
KNEES SWING:	L	L	L	L	L	L	L	L

ARMS: Swing around in RIGHT (C.W.) circle on EVERY count!

You can swing the knees RIGHT on every count by circling the arms LEFT!

SHIFT:

COUNT:	1 2 3 4	&	5 6 7 8	&	1 2 3 4	&	5 6 7 8	&
KNEES GO:	L R L R	L	R L R L	R	L R L R	L	R L R L	R
MEASURE:	Left——		Right——		Left——		Right——	
ARMS SWING:	R L R L	R	L R L R	L	R L R L	R	L R L R	L
PATTERN:	Left Basic	*	Right Reverse Basic	*	Left Basic	*	Right Reverse Basic	*

* The "AND" count is the EXTRA SWING that makes the "SHIFT" from the BASIC to the REVERSE BASIC and back.

Done from either BASIC or SIDE BASIC position, the Shift consists of doing one measure accenting the DOWNBEAT to the left — followed by one measure accenting the DOWNBEAT to the RIGHT! In order to connect the two, an "and" count shifts the position for the next measure*.

One of the "fun things" about TWIST is being able to play games with your partner. You will see everythig from cowboys throwing a rope and pulling the girl in — to the old "bug bit" where one partner throws an imaginary bug at his partner and the "chase" provides the entertainment. Let YOUR imagination play games. Remember that dancing should be fun, but not ridiculous. No matter WHICH dance you are doing, the most important part will be the basic motion and rhythm. Concentrate on these two things FIRST. Variations are easy things to learn AFTER the basics become second nature.

1978 Comment . . . The above paragraph could have been written TODAY! The BODY LANGUAGE is using all kinds of "BITS" that are as individual as the Dancers care to be.

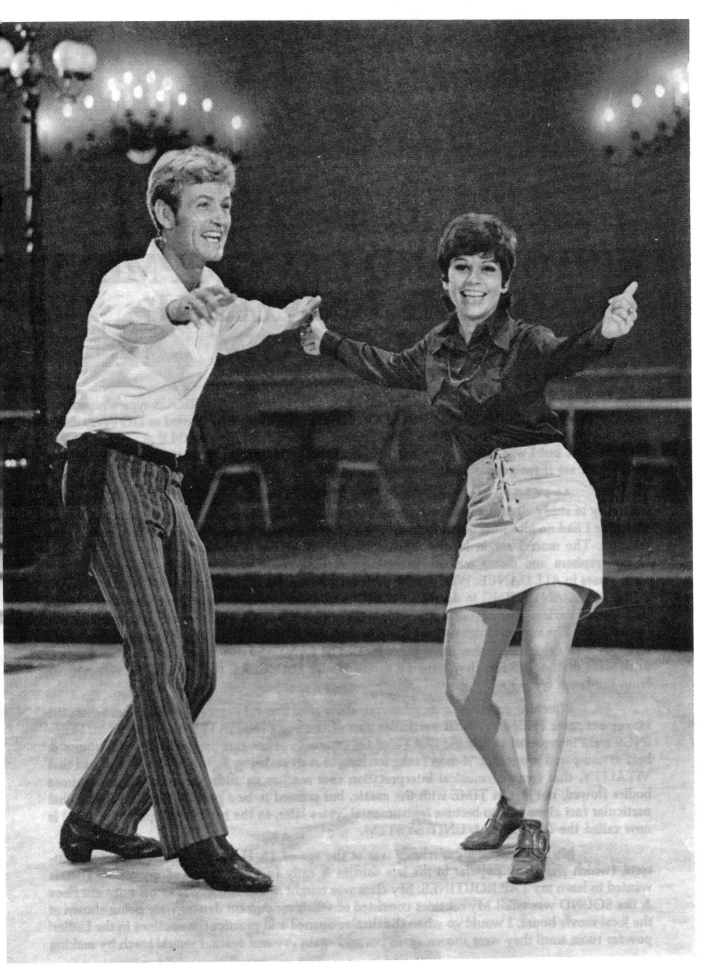

Chapter X

HISTORY AND DEVELOPMENT OF THE UNIVERSAL UNIT SYSTEM

From the time I was a small child, I have always been the CURIOUS type who wanted to know WHY? . . . HOW? . . . & CAN I DO THAT TOO? I not only wanted to DO every dance that I saw performed ala ASTAIRE AND ROGERS . . . or SHIRLEY TEMPLE . . . or ELEANOR POWELL . . . but I was interested in the MOVEMENT, TIMING & MUSICAL INTERPRETATION that set these people apart from the crowd.

As a Child performer on the STEEL PIER in Atlantic City, New Jersey, I had the opportunity to study all of the vaudeville performers that appeared on that magnificent stage. . . . At that time I had no idea how much influence this early training would have on the future of Dance training. The more I sat in on the rehearsals of some of the big shows, observing the master choreographers and dance trainers in action, teaching their performers, the more I saw the samenesses in ALL DANCE. Whether the performance was by a Ballet Dancer, a Ballroom Dancer, a Juggler . . . ANYTHING to do with MUSIC AND MOVEMENT . . . There was a correlation that seemed to flow thru my mind that ALL MOVEMENT is ONE. The common denominator was the MUSIC. The way in which each of these performers interpreted the music and particularly the RHYTHM of the music, either made them look to be FANTASTIC dancers, AVERAGE dancers, or dancers that looked like they were TRYING TO BE DANCERS. (SOMETHING was missing from the latter types.)

Watching rehearsal after rehearsal, show after show, I came to be able to see where the movement came FROM . . . what particular part of the body INITIATED the movement. FEELINGS were interpreted to specific BEATS of the music. . . . How one person interpreted sound & beat as compared to another. It didn't take too long to start realizing that the dancers who had that VITALITY, that sense of musical interpretation that reaches an audience were the ones whose bodies flowed, not just in TIME with the music, but seemed to be a part OF THE MUSIC. That particular fact alone was to become instrumental, years later, in the basic development of what is now called the UNIVERSAL UNIT SYSTEM.

My first teaching experience was at the age of 13. Having won many amateur contests, (which were very popular in the late thirties & early forties), several of my school friends wanted to learn my TAP ROUTINES. My class was taught in our BASEMENT on a cement floor & the SOUND was wild! My routines consisted of whatever current dances were being shown at the local movie house. I would go when the theater opened and practice the routines in the Ladies' powder room until they were shown again . . . and again . . . and again. I would teach by making clicking sounds, verbally, to the music . . . that accented the various rhythms. Later, in order to have something for the students to refer to, in order to remember the routine, I put down these little "clicking" sounds by VERBAL COUNT, "ta tum, ta tum, ta ta ta tum." At that time, I would leave a space between the sounds to indicate MEASURES OF MUSIC.

In HIGH SCHOOL I wrote a lot of PLAYS and MUSIC and choreographed Dances that went with the music. The routines were taught, using the TA TUM sound system. Having observed that in the SCHOOL DANCE CLASSES, the teacher counted STEPS, rather than BEATS of music, I also became aware that a LARGE NUMBER OF STUDENTS could NOT KEEP TIME TO MUSIC when they were not dancing WITH the teacher's assistance. NOR could they dance the same material to OTHER MUSIC. At the same time that these classes were going on, I was producing a MUSICAL, using some of the same dancers. In order to correct the TIMING problem I kept everything to the actual MUSICAL COUNT, rather than the STEPS. I am sure that many of the BETTER TEACHERS of the day were already counting BEATS instead of STEPS, but the personal discovery (not having had the advantage of formal training at that time) . . . the personal discovery of SEEING the DIFFERENCE when one was counting steps . . . & another counting BEATS, made a lasting impression & was to become of paramount importance in the development of the UNIVERSAL UNIT SYSTEM. The young people who were in those shows . . . & were exposed to the breaking up of the EIGHT COUNTS were always ON TIME and could do these same sequences to any piece of music with a similar rhythm. At that time, because we were doing so many DIFFERENT shows, I developed a little language which I could use to take PIECES of patterns . . . take ONE OF THESE and ONE OF THOSE and rearrange them into another routine.

Some of these dancers got to be able to do this so well, that they went on to do their own choreography . . . and several of them became professional dancers.

My GOAL at that particular time was to WRITE and PRODUCE my own musicals. The DANCE was important to me, but the WRITING and DIRECTING was more important.

In the early forties, JITTERBUG, or SWING as we know it today, was THE most important social dance of the day. On the STEEL PIER in ATLANTIC CITY, there were many CONTESTS and SWING DANCES. (We danced to every top name in the BIG BAND field.) Because young men in the service came from all over the country, the VARIETY of styles was wide. Many of the girl dancers were confined to the particular style that they knew. I had a particular eye for noting the SAMENESSES of the RHYTHM, but noting the ALTERATION of the lead. Being able to observe both the SAMENESSES and the DIFFERENCES of RHYTHM and STYLE allowed me to adjust my dancing to ANY partner. This SOCIAL aspect of the dance was to become far more important to me than any of us could have realized at the time.

It wasn't until TEN YEARS, one wonderful husband, and four lovely children later that my interest in DANCING surfaced again, laying the foundation for the current text. It was then that I attended TEACHERS TRAINING for a National Chain Studio, under the capable direction of JERRY ERHARDT. Jerry had his hands full in that most of the participants in that training class were ALREADY dancers of one kind or another. Some were SWING CONTESTANTS, some were TAP DANCERS, one was an ACROBAT from a circus . . . and of the twelve who graduated (some 35 or more started), eight eventually owned their own studios or became professional dancers in the entertainment field. Jerry counts that class as his best effort and we all loved him. I taught for that school for three years and was continually disturbed by the fact that more emphasis was placed on the SELLING of a course, than on the TEACHING of the lesson. The PHRASE was "SELL THE SIZZLE and not the STEAK." My analytical mind was more interested in THE STEAK! Their reasoning, and I am sure it was a valid one, was that if the salesman did not SELL the course, the Teacher would have no students to teach. I am sure that these modes of operation are a service to the students whom they serve. However, my particular interest in dance WAS, and IS, for the MASSES. My analytical mind saw ALL DANCE as ONE and was eager to devise a system whereby communication was possible in the DIFFERENT MEDIUMS of the DANCE.

Anyone involved in DANCE of any form, has met with the lack of communication of one form to another. Ballet dancers do not consider SOCIAL DANCERS as dancers. A MODERN

JAZZ DANCER does not feel the relationship to SQUARE DANCING or FOLK DANCING. A SWING DANCER does not usually relate to WALTZ . . . and yet that one common denominator, . . . the MUSIC, the BEAT of the music seemed to me to be the linking factor to ALL DANCE.

It was in 1959 that I decided to open my own school of dance, for the sole purpose of proving that the CONCEPT that I had in my mind would produce knowledgable dancers, in all fields, in less time than had been the usual custom. My GOAL for the studio was to perfect a system whereby the STUDENT was not limited by the capabilities of the TEACHER:

. . . A great NOVELIST did not necessarily have a great ENGLISH TEACHER, but he was given the TOOLS with which to first COPY . . . and then CREATE.

. . . A great COMPOSER was not confined by the limitations of his music teacher. He learned how to use the TOOLS. He was given basic RULES and the concepts on which those rules were founded.

. . . A sound SYSTEM OF LEARNING must have sound RULES and sound BASICS from which to build. I felt that I had discovered the COMMON DENOMINATOR for ALL DANCE and the opening of the SKIPPY BLAIR STUDIOS in DOWNEY, CALIFORNIA was the beginning of twenty years of RESEARCH, DEVELOPMENT and plain HARD WORK, to prove my theories.

The Studio grew from ONE building to FOUR buildings in its fifteen years of operation. During that period of time, not only SOCIAL CLASSES and PERFORMING ARTS CLASSES were developed, but there were special classes for the mentally retarded, STUDIED RELAXATION Classes, MOTION STUDY CLASSES, Summer WORKSHOPS and continuous TEACHERS TRAINING CLASSES. During those fifteen years, many of my personal students were recommended to me by DOCTORS, PSYCHOLOGISTS and PSYCHIATRISTS . . . and the DANCE and particularly the TEACHING OF THE DANCE became more closely entwined, to me, with the DEVELOPMENT OF HUMAN POTENTIAL (See Chapter for "Teachers Only").

During the early stages of the studio, our STUDENTS and our TEACHERS WON OR PLACED in almost every competition that they entered. (Our people are still doing that today!)

DANCE COMPETITIONS serve a necessary purpose in the DANCE WORLD in that they provide an incentive for a certain percentage of dancers to perfect their craft. However, my particular interest is NOT in the competition of ONE PERSON against ANOTHER but rather helping each person to REACH HIS OR HER OWN POTENTIAL. Each person, ideally, should only be in competition with HIMSELF. (See chapter on COMPETITION & PERFORMANCE.) The only purpose in mentioning competition at this point, was to show that THE SYSTEM was working. The difference between our dancers and other dancers was described in various ways. Some described it as having more "Class" . . . others said "STYLE" . . . but I knew the secret was in THE SYSTEM.

In 1963 I published my first Dance Text Book entitled "SO YOU WANT TO LEARN TO DANCE?" The limited edition of 500 copies was for the purpose of FEEDBACK before publishing a book for students. The 1963 publication was primarily for teachers who had been trained in the UNIVERSAL UNIT SYSTEM, to aid them in their teaching and to have a handy reference book at their fingertips. As a teacher's aid it was tremendously successful for those WHO HAD HAD SPECIFIC TRAINING IN THE SYSTEM, but was too complicated for the average new teacher. It was DEFINITELY too complicated for students. (As complicated as it was for some, we still get comments from teachers who consider the 1963 version one of the most up-to-date and relevant text books in their library.)

The NEXT STAGE OF DEVELOPMENT in the UNIVERSAL UNIT SYSTEM is one that should be a lesson to all of us in every stage of life. In looking for ways to SIMPLIFY the system, I steadfastly held on to those ideas which I had been taught . . . as TRUTH. I had ADDED to what I had learned, but never thought of CHANGING COMPLETELY that which I held to be TRUTH.

All of the accepted systems of SOCIAL DANCE . . . (including the one that I had learned) had a series of RHYTHMS that were interchangebable in the dancing of SWING. Some used those same rhythms for MAMBO and some of the other RHYTHM DANCES. Those rhythms were . . . and please note this carefully:

SINGLE RHYTHM . . . referred to as TWO BEATS, stepping on the first and holding or touching on the second (ONE WEIGHT CHANGE.)

TRIPLE RHYTHM . . . which stepped THREE TIMES to TWO BEATS of music, either Left right left . . . or Right left right.

. . . and then DOUBLE RHYTHM . . . which for some unknown reason, held the first beat of music and stepped on the second beat (tap STEP).

This particular system was merely an interchange of rhythms, but not a COMPLETE SYSTEM because there was NO RHYTHM for STEPPING TWICE. My 1963 book KEPT the RHYTHMS intact as they are stated above, because I accepted them as FACT. I ADDED a RHYTHM that stepped TWICE and called it a COMBINATION UNIT.

For years, students had been experiencing difficulty with DOUBLE RHYTHM, and I shudder to think HOW MANY TIMES someone asked, "WHY DOESN'T DOUBLE RHYTHM STEP TWICE?" . . . Teachers all over the country would patiently explain any one of a large assortment of reasons that somehow convinced the student that DOUBLE RHYTHM did indeed only step one time, on the second count of music. My COMBINATION UNIT (stepping two times to two beats of music), along with the accepted SINGLE, DOUBLE and TRIPLE RHYTHMS made a COMPLETE SYSTEM applicable to ALL dance. It was STILL too complicated for the average student.

Secure in the knowledge that there is an ANSWER to EVERY PROBLEM, I taught experimental classes, teachers sessions, the mentally retarded . . . any situation that I thought might bring me closer to what I knew was a reality: That there IS an UNCOMPLICATED, basic foundation to ALL DANCE . . . and that I held the key to the answer in my UNIVERSAL UNIT SYSTEM.*

What seemed like a catastrophe turned out to be a BLESSING. The PURPOSE in opening the STUDIO in Downey, was to perfect the UNIT SYSTEM and to prove out the system by training teachers and dancers. I had done that to my own and everyone else's satisfaction. Now, some of my teachers had become professional dancers. Two were headlining in Las Vegas. One was in Puerto Rico. One had opened his own school in Northern California. The NEED for the Studio was no longer there. I needed to get on with the business of "Spreading the Word" and very little time was being spent in the Studio itself. Most of my classes were OUTSIDE the Studio: Schools, Parks, Teachers' Seminars, at other Studios and Out of State . . . and the HUGE CLASSES that had developed at the GOLDEN WEST BALLROOM in Norwalk. Then . . . THE CATASTROPHE . . . I injured my back and the verdict was COMPRESSED DISC . . . MUST OPERATE . . . will be out of Studio for six months to a year.

Could this be true? I had prayed for an answer as to how to terminate the Studio so that I would be free to do the things I wanted to do . . . But wasn't this a bit of a drastic solution? Feeling that the exercises and postures that I had been teaching would suffice to see me thru this dilemma, I vetoed the operation and decided to see the pain thru. (A public thank you to those dear friends who saw me thru that traumatic period.) Needless to say, I closed the Studio. My personal PHILOSOPHY OF LIFE is that WHAT SEEMS TO BE A NEGATIVE . . . IS ALWAYS A POSITIVE IN DISGUISE. It is only our PERCEPTION that gives us momentary doubt.

Fortunately, I had well trained teachers who took over for me at the GOLDEN WEST BALLROOM. Meantime, flat on my back, I had many hours to MEDITATE, to think about the UNIT SYSTEM, THE BOOK, THE FUTURE. Little by little I was able to start my YOGA POSTURES and develop strength in the spine. After six weeks I was able to teach one hour a day. Later, I could handle two hours a day. Meantime, there were many hours of concentrated thought and Meditation. I knew it was for a purpose. The ANSWERS to every question are within our grasp. Sometimes we just don't take time to FIND THEM. I now had TIME and I knew the answers were close at hand.

While searching for the ANSWER to making the system less complicated, I came across an article on creativity that stated that we sometimes overlook the OBVIOUS because we accept PRIOR KNOWLEDGE AS FACT. I also came across the statement that in looking for answers, we "LIMIT THE ANSWERS BY THE LIMITATION OF OUR QUESTIONS." I gave that considerable thought and reasoned that my PROBLEM lay in the ORIGINAL SET OF RHYTHM VARIATIONS . . . Back to the DRAWING BOARD, my thought traveled to the fact that if you can't teach the BASICS to an eight year old, your system is too complicated. . . . SIMPLIFY . . . SIMPLIFY . . . SIMPLIFY . . . The key word to all teaching.

The following day, an eight year old in a DAY SCHOOL CLASS, eager to tell me how much she was learning, gave me the KEY that would finally put the pieces of the puzzle in place. I had just explained SINGLE RHYTHM and TRIPLE RHYTHM and the children had performed the exercises to music. (I always taught DOUBLE RHYTHM last because it was the hardest to explain.) Before I got that far, this new little girl said, "Teacher, teacher . . . I know . . . If Single Rhythm steps ONCE and Triple Rhythm steps 3 Times then DOUBLE RHYTHM MUST STEP TWICE!" (How many times had I heard that before but NEVER REALLY HEARD?) I get goose bumps even now, recalling the excitement of DISCOVERY. The answer had been there all along. That moment opened the door to the current SIMPLIFIED SYSTEM. I told that little girl that she was absolutely correct, and proceeded to teach the class based on that premise. It was one of the most exciting classes I have ever taught. The children responded exceptionally well and all of the pieces seemed to fall into place. It was now 1972.

Up until this time (as in the 1963 book) the UNITS were oblong boxes that contained descriptions of steps. Each BOX was TWO BEATS OF MUSIC. Each BOX was a UNIT. They were written out for each pattern like this:

STEP TOUCH	TAP STEP	STEP THREE TIMES	STEP STEP

Again . . . the system WORKED, but was not GRAPHIC enough. Now that I had made the decision that DOUBLE RHYTHM WOULD STEP TWICE, I was faced with explaining to my constituents that I was CHANGING A RHYTHM THAT WAS KNOWN WORLD-WIDE TO BE SOMETHING OTHER THAN WHAT I SAID IT WAS. It was not an easy decision. It is NEVER easy to admit that there is a BETTER WAY and that what I knew YESTERDAY might be OBSOLETE today. For my OWN USE, I had developed a sort of SHORT HAND using DOTS AND SLASHES. Here was my GRAPHIC ANSWER. I enclosed my DOTS AND SLASHES in long skinny BOXES and the UNIT CARDS WERE BORN. They now looked like this:

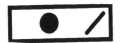 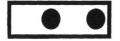 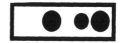 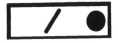

SINGLE RHYTHM   DOUBLE RHYTHM   TRIPLE RHYTHM   DELAYED SINGLE

HOW VERY SIMPLE IT ALL SEEMED. WHY HADN'T SOMEONE DONE THIS BEFORE? STEP ONCE . . . STEP TWICE . . . STEP THREE TIMES. Surely there must be a CATCH somewhere. I went carefully over EVERY BASIC STEP in EVERY DANCE and found they could be done using JUST THOSE THREE PRIMARY UNITS. Even though many of our teachers had used the UNIT SYSTEM for their own use, very few had found it advantageous to use it with students. NOW, ALL OF A SUDDEN . . . THE UNIT CARDS and the SIMPLIFICATION OF RHYTHMS made DANCE HISTORY . . . Requests came from all over when the word got out. Teachers made their own UNIT CARDS and several different styles were tried. The RESULT is the dimension that you see in this book.

The SKIPPY BLAIR DANCE EXPERIENCE NOTEBOOK was published in 1973/1974, explaining the SYSTEM and how to TEACH IT. It did not include PATTERNS. Much of the material in that book has been revised and is included in this one.

That period from 1973 thru 1978 has been a demanding one. The UNIVERSAL UNIT SYSTEM has spread far and wide. The reports from TEACHERS IN THE COLLEGES are numerous. With the closing of the Studio, the GOLDEN WEST BALLROOM became headquarters for the GOLDEN STATE DANCE ASSOCIATION and our sincere thanks go to OLEN THIBIDEAU, owner of the Ballroom, who supported our TEACHERS' SESSIONS and has been instrumental in furthering DANCE EDUCATION by making special arrangements with the COLLEGE STUDENTS AND TEACHERS for them to attend the classes at the Ballroom. At this writing, September 1978, all of my efforts for the past twenty-five years have been condensed and refined to help YOU become a BETTER DANCER. I hand YOU the KEYS. Use them well and you will reap the benefits for the rest of your life.

The DANCE EDUCATION AND INFORMATION BUREAU, a non-profit corporation dedicated to PROGRESS IN THE DEVELOPMENT OF HUMAN POTENTIAL is interested in YOUR reaction and progress thru the system. Your responses are welcome.

Sincerely, Yours for better dancing,

Skippy Blair

𝔊olden 𝔖tate 𝔇ance 𝔗eachers 𝔄ssn.
10804 Woodruff Ave.   Downey, CA 90241
www.swingworld.com   562-869-8949

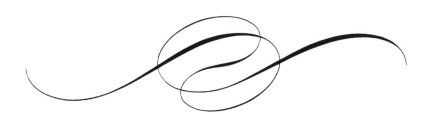

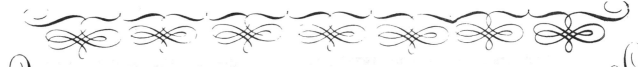

AMERICA'S DANCING
HALL OF FAME

THIS AWARD PRESENTED TO

Skippy Blair

UPON BEING INDUCTED INTO
THE HALL OF FAME
FOR UNSELFISH AND DEVOTED SERVICE
TO AMERICAN DANCING
AUGUST 12, 1978

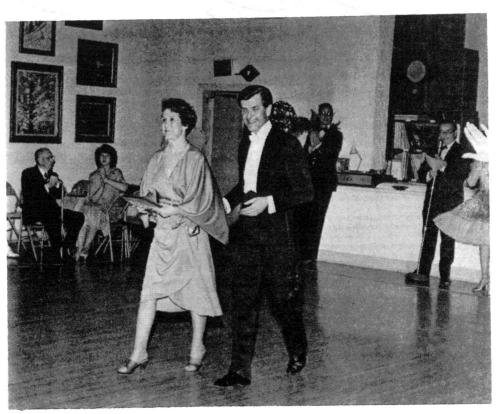

ANOTHER — "Picture from the Past" 1960 "SKIPPY BLAIR DANC-
ERS at DISNEYLAND" The Summer Dance Competition and show
filled the Pavillion every Wednesday night.

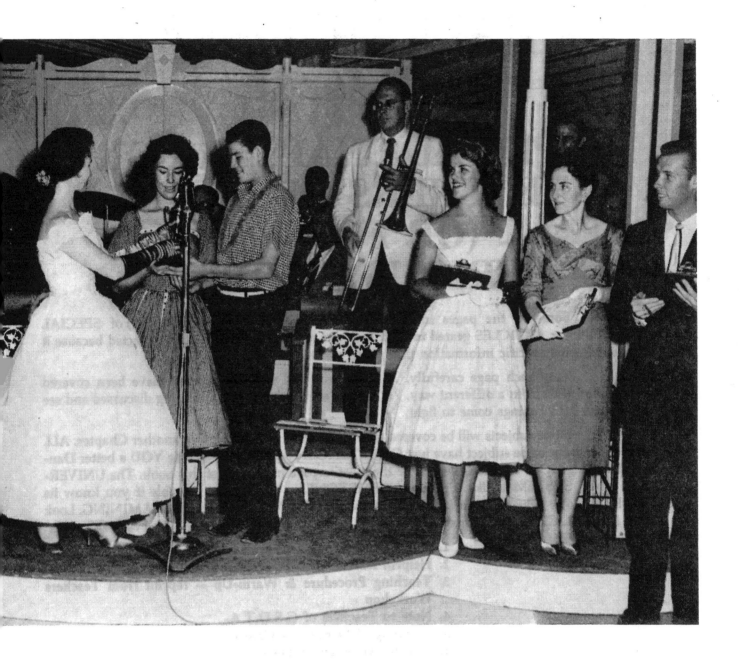

Pictured from L to R: Skippy Blair, Teenage couple, BILL ELLIOTT &
Elliott Bros. orchestra, BARBARA BOYLAN (Bobby Burgess' 1st
partner on Lawrence Welk show), CHLOE CALL of Call's Fine Arts,
and JOHN BUCKNER, G.S.D.T.A. Barbara, Chloe and John were fre-
quent judges.

Chapter XI

SPECIAL CHAPTER FOR TEACHERS OF DANCE (OR FOR THE SERIOUS STUDENT)

Some of the pages in this Chapter are made up of REPRINTS of SPECIAL BULLETINS or ARTICLES geared toward Teachers of Dance. Each has been selected because it contained some specific information that might not appear elsewhere.

Read each page carefully. . . . You will find some points that have been covered before, but perhaps in a different way. . . . Reflect on the specific points being discussed and see how many NEW things come to light.

Some subjects will be covered from a different point of view in another Chapter. ALL aproaches to the same subject have just ONE THING IN MIND. . . . Making YOU a better Dancer! Learning HOW to LEARN is one of the most important aspects of this book. The UNIVERSAL UNIT SYSTEM is like a precious GEMSTONE. . . . It is only valuable if you know its WORTH. To be valuable, it requires POLISHING . . . EXAMINING and RE-EXAMINING. Look at it in ALL LIGHTS. . . . Learn every facet . . . and its value will increase with every exposure.

Included:
1. Rules Versus Tools — reprint from Teachers Workshop
2. Helpful Rules of U.U.S. — reprint from Teachers Workshop
3. Teaching Procedure & Warm-Up — reprint from Teachers Workshop
4. Note to Teachers of G.S.D.T.A.
5. Teaching of Dance as a Career
6. Holistic Approach to Dance
7. 3 most frequently asked questions
   re: Universal Unit System

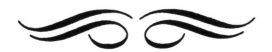

RULES versus TOOLS

"Rules are those things which ALWAYS APPLY ... A RULE is a TRUTH ... A TOOL is something we use to FIX things. We constantly CHANGE our tools according to the need. RULES remain the same."

The purpose of the above paragraph is to answer the many teachers who have devised teaching "TOOLS" and ask if they must be abandoned with the UNIT SYSTEM. NO ... definitely NOT! Teaching Tools are those things we use to better explain a particular action to a SPECIFIC PERSON. The RULE may not have been clear. The TOOL is one to get that particular person to do that which we are trying to teach. ...

> Example: Mary has been told that in order to improve her dancing her spine should be erect, and her head held high. Mary tilts her head BACK and her hips are pushed back also.

> The TEACHER tells Mary to "pull her chin down" and to "push her hips forward." These are NOT RULES ... only TOOLS to get Mary to achieve the RULE.

... Someone else LISTENING to what is being said, comes away saying that we should dance with our CHINS PULLED DOWN ... AND OUR HIPS PUSHED FORWARD. CLARIFY when you use a TOOL to achieve a certain result. Be AWARE of the effect on the rest of the class ... or on the future thinking of the individual in question.

> RULES are those things which we put in print ... those things which we can count on to be consistent ... those things which form the foundation.

> TOOLS are the things we devise to correct a fault.

Try to use more RULES, than TOOLS. Go back to the BASIC FUNDAMENTALS OF TEACHING. Does the student know:

> ... The RHYTHM STRUCTURE OF THE PATTERN ?
> ... How many UNITS in the pattern ?
> ... The DIRECTION and FOOT POSITIONS in the pattern ?
> ... The DIRECTION of the CENTER POINT OF BALANCE ?
> ... The specific LEAD for the pattern ?
> ... The Basic MOVEMENT and characteristic of the dance ?

Chances are that you will need less and less teaching TOOLS as you use the rules of the system. However, improvisation has always been the key-word to good teaching. The UNIT SYSTEM should give you even MORE freedom to create ... and to grow. It should in no way inhibit your teaching.

Golden State Dance Teachers Association

REPRINT
1977

Compiled for TEACHERS TRAINING. December 1977
Revised April 1993

HELPFUL RULES OF THE UNIVERSAL UNIT SYSTEM

1. Knowing the actual SEPARATE BODY UNITS and RHYTHM UNITS, and not just the number of weight changes in a complete pattern, will make it easy to UNDERSTAND the components of the Dance.

2. ....Count the actual BEATS of MUSIC in a complete pattern. Do NOT count.... "ONE TWO THREE...ONE TWO THREE." The first ONE TWO THREE would not be the same as the next ONE TWO THREE. If the pattern has FOUR beats of music, and is composed of two TRIPLES, the count would be "ONE & TWO and THREE & FOUR."

3. There is NO time when the feet should not be in a CORRECT FOOT POSITION. Every pattern has correct foot positions for EVERY STEP. If someone takes your picture in the middle of a turn and catches you in an awkward pose, the fault does NOT lie with the timing of the photographer. KNOW which position makes each pattern work.

4. Unless otherwise specified, the Lady will always be dancing a "Natural Opposite" in a couples dance.

5. All series of patterns (Amalgamations) should begin at the beginning of a PHRASE.

6. The "CALL" for a specific pattern should be "CALLED" on the Unit BEFORE the pattern starts. (See Line Dances for Exceptions.)

7. An EVEN UNIT can be substituted for any other EVEN UNIT to add RHYTHM VARIATIONS to almost any Dance.

8. An ODD UNIT can be substituted for any other ODD UNIT to add RHYTHM VARIATIONS to almost any Dance.

9. The CENTER POINT OF BALANCE is the DRIVING FORCE and RECEIVING FORCE, (Action and Reaction) that creates the look of ONENESS that is necessary to fully appreciate Couples Dancing. The Man's LEAD should be an EXTENSION of his OWN C.P.B. The leverage is not achieved with pushing, pulling, heel of the hand, fingertips, etc. . . . but by the natural movement of his OWN C.P.B.

10. ALL DANCE (Social Dance in particular) contains some degree of VERTICAL MOVEMENT. What APPEARS to the untrained eye as HORIZONTAL movement is actually VERTICAL MOVEMENT that has been S T R E T C H ED out. The PRESS into the floor that creates the body projection is the SAME PRESS to move UPWARD as it is to move OUTWARD. The degree of movement in a particular direction determines the amount of VISIBLE movement.

14. Isolate the BASIC MOVEMENT of each Dance before attempting to do the patterns. . . . Practice that movement to Music.

15. The FREE FOOT is just as important as the WEIGHTED FOOT. Be aware of the Movement and Control of the FREE FOOT.

16. To make the transition from partners dancing OPPOSITE FOOT to partners dancing SAME FOOT, one partner (usually the man) will substitute an EVEN UNIT for an ODD UNIT . . . or an ODD UNIT for an EVEN UNIT. To return to the former position, the same substitution is repeated.

17. A ONE UNIT or TWO UNIT "LINK" can be used to join patterns together to make them PHRASE.

18. Any pattern can be EXTENDED by adding a DOUBLE RHYTHM UNIT. (No matter how many DOUBLE RHYTHM UNITS are added, the same foot will be free.)

19. Any BASIC RHYTHM UNIT can be extended by adding TWO STEPS. An EXTENDED DOUBLE steps FOUR TIMES to Two beats of Music. An EXTENDED TRIPLE steps FIVE TIMES to Two beats of Music. We do not extend a SINGLE RHYTHM UNIT because it would become a TRIPLE.

20. All DANCE PATTERNS (with the exception of WALTZ) will consist of an EVEN NUMBER OF BEATS. Knowing the UNITS that comprise the Pattern assures the correct count. We hear of the SEVEN STEP or the FIVE STEP pattern and we know immediately that someone is counting STEPS instead of BEATS OF MUSIC. This leads to dancing OUT OF TIME WITH THE MUSIC.

"To be able to develop a student to HIS own highest potential, and not confine him to our own capabilities. . . . THAT should be the sincere goal of every Teacher."

. . . Skippy Blair . . .

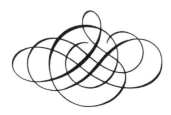

TEACHING PROCEDURE:

1. Establish the UNIT STRUCTURE OF THE PATTERN:

   A. How many UNITS in the PATTERN? . . . What KIND?

   B. Clap out or STEP out the RHYTHM PATTERN. (STEP TWICE/STEP THREE TIMES etc.)

   C. STEP OUT THE RHYTHM as you COUNT the BEATS OF MUSIC.

2. Add DIRECTION with the FOOT POSITIONS in EACH UNIT

3. Add appropriate TURNS or ANGLES involving CENTER POINT OF BALANCE.

   A. Where is the C.P.B. aiming?

4. Add BASIC MOVEMENT if any . . . or appropriate DRIVE.

   A. Does this dance require a BOUNCING UNIT? . . . a DRIVING UNIT?

5. Clarify the LEADS, along with DANCE POSITION

6. Put it all together to THE MUSIC!!

Ask of your STUDENT, your CLASS, or YOURSELF, the following questions about EACH PATTERN that you learn:

1. How many UNITS in the PATTERN ?

2. What is the "VERBAL" PATTERN ?
   ("Forward/Forward/Side Together Side") etc.

3. What are the FOOT POSITIONS in the KEY UNITS ?

4. What is the ESSENCE of the Dance ?

THE "WARM-UP" . . .

In PERFORMING ARTS CLASSES (Tap, Ballet, Jazz etc.) there is always a Warm-Up that conditions your body for movement . . . and your mind for learning. In SOCIAL DANCE, a WARM-UP serves the same purpose.

Practice the INDIVIDUAL UNITS in different directions, keeping time to MUSIC. It doesn't take long before your feet start responding automatically when the music starts. CALL OUT the individual UNITS as they are danced:

"LEFT SINGLE . . . RIGHT SINGLE" . . . Do this "touching in FIRST FOOT POSITION . . . then touching in an extended FIFTH FOOT POSITION . . . then do it by KICKING FORWARD instead of a TOUCH.

"LEFT TRIPLE . . . RIGHT TRIPLE" . . . Do your TRIPLES starting with a Side Together Side (to the Left and to the Right.) . . . Then moving Forward and Backward in THIRD FOOT POSITION, and in FOURTH FOOT POSITION.

"DOUBLE RHYTHM . . . DOUBLE RHYTHM" . . . March in Place . . . Then March with One foot FORWARD and One foot BACK . . . Then try "SIDE TOGETHERS" around the room. Repeat all the DOUBLE RHYTHM, starting on the other foot.

Golden State Dance Teachers Association

REPRINT

May 22, 1978

Special Note to: Teachers of the UNIVERSAL UNIT SYSTEM working for or in conjunction with The Golden State Dance Teachers Association.

1. Lessons should be FUN . . . EXCITING . . . and still RELAXED and COMFORTABLE.

2. Students should be made to feel that it is YOUR RESPONSIBILITY to teach them.

3. The lesson should begin with a quick but thorough WARM-UP including all of the Basic RHYTHM VARIATIONS plus the FOOT POSITIONS that you plan to teach for that particular lesson.

4. The lesson should end on a HIGH NOTE. Always end with something that has been a complete success for EVERYONE. A FOLLOW THE LEADER circle to an UP TEMPO will end the class on a high note. Make sure that everything you do is EASY TO DO and done to EASY MUSIC with a STRONG BEAT.

5. PLAN YOUR LESSON. Know the G.S.D.T.A. Curriculum for what you are teaching. Doing YOUR OWN THING may be acceptable in an emergency, but on a continuing basis even the STUDENTS will know the difference. Today's students are an educated audience. Do not insult their intelligence.

6. The reputation of the G.S.D.T.A. has been founded on 20 years of excellence in the field of Dance. Make sure that you are CONTRIBUTING to that reputation and not being responsible for any letdown as we grow.

7. Don't be afraid to ASK QUESTIONS. When something goes wrong in class . . . or you are having problems with a particular student . . . PRESENT YOUR PROBLEM . . . and get the answer. The UNIVERSAL UNIT SYSTEM is a COMPLETE SYSTEM of learning. When you are having problems ONE OF THE PROCEDURES is probably being overlooked!

8. Be aware of EVERY STUDENT IN THE CLASS. In "backing up" to explain something for one person . . . you will probably clarify that same thing for many more.

9. USE THE TERMINOLOGY. Count out the actual beats of music in a pattern. Also refer to the actual UNITS in the pattern. Use the FOOT POSITIONS by name for clarification of a particular stance or move. REFER TO C.P.B. (Center Point of Balance) whenever applicable. Refer to the BASIC MOVEMENT UNIT when applicable. Know the KEY UNIT in a pattern and teach it separately. Know the FORCE POINT of specific moves of the hands or feet and USE THE TERMINOLOGY!

10. Conduct your class as if everyone there would have to take an examination. Know the BASIC things that your student should cover in order to PASS an examination. Ask questions of the class or student that will tell you what they DO know and what they do NOT know.

11. PHRASE out the music that you plan to teach to. Always start in TIME with the music. Always start at the beginning of a MEASURE. The "CALL" should be on the UNIT prior to the start of the MEASURE. Starting on the HEAVY MEASURE is preferable but any measure is acceptable. Starting in the MIDDLE of the measure, even though it is the beginning of a Unit is an UNCOMFORTABLE spot to start. It will eventually TRAIN OUT the ability to hear minor phrases. Starting on the HEAVY MEASURE will train the ear to hear phrasing.

Golden State Dance Teachers Association

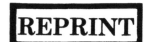

Cal State Fullerton Career Day, April 21, 1978

THE TEACHING OF DANCE AS A CAREER OR AN AVOCATION

Never before in the History of Dance have there been so many opportunities for employment in this particular field. There are so many different areas to explore that one can literally "take their pick" and find success IF they choose carefully and prepare themselves thoroughly.

- PERFORMING ARTS: In the area of BALLET . . . TAP DANCING . . . MODERN JAZZ and more recently JAZZ DISCO, the entire country is turned on to the sense of accomplishment that comes with being able to perform. The physical and mental discipline that comes with weekly or sometimes daily training is fast becoming an alternative to other, less creative forms of exercise. From Pre-schoolers to Senior Citizens . . . and all ages in between, there are more and more people in need of qualified instruction. As leisure time increases, the need grows.

   Studios, Parks and Recreation, Schools both Private and Public are in need of QUALIFIED Teachers. The Area of PERFORMING ARTS expands yearly. Info: DANCE INFORMATION BUREAU (213) 869-7510.

- DANCE THERAPY: There is a growing field of DANCE THERAPISTS in the Dance community. Dance Therapy has been with us for many years, but is just now becoming publicized enough for others to become aware of their existence. The DANCE ANALYST is in a unique position in that many times the "patient" is unaware that treatment is taking place. Therefore the normal resistance to change and growth that usually exists in other forms of therapy are eliminated in the Dance. This is an exciting field for those who have a genuine interest in the development of human potential.

   Information will be sent, by inquiring through ADTA (American Dance Therapy Association) Suite #230, 2000 Century Plaza, Columbia, Maryland 21044. Phone: (301) 997-4040. Local therapists may be reached through the DANCE INFORMATION BUREAU (213) 869-7510.

- SOCIAL DANCE (TRADITIONAL and/or CONTEMPORARY): Social Dance today is in an awakening period that will last for many years. Even when the current excitement levels out, the demand will still be great. Everyone from 5th Grade to Senior Citizen wants to "LEARN TO DANCE."

   Actors and Actresses are frequently called upon to portray personalities which require the SOCIAL DANCE of a particular era. The era of the late seventies will be known throughout history as the Renaissance of Social Dance. Following a period of almost extinction of Social Dance, there was a five year period of isolating "movement without form." (It must be noted here that through ALL CHANGING PERIODS, the traditional social dance groups had their own Dance Community complete with Competitions, etc.) Here, we speak of SOCIAL DANCE in the context of the average AMERICAN ADULT. TODAY . . . The AVERAGE AMERICAN ADULT is involved in SOME FORM of SOCIAL DANCE. The Dance has come full circle. TANGO HUSTLE/ LATIN HUSTLE/ CHA CHA/ SWING/ CALIFORNIA SHUFFLE/ SALSA/ Yesterday's Dances Reborn.

The UNIVERSAL UNIT SYSTEM is a relatively new concept in the teaching of Dance. Although it has been around since 1963, the System has been used almost exclusively for training TEACHERS until 1971 when the UNIVERSAL UNIT SYSTEM became the standard examination for the GOLDEN STATE DANCE TEACHERS ASSOCIATION. Since that time, the System has been used for all forms of DANCE TRAINING starting with Pre-School Children, up through College Classes. Employment opportunities are unlimited for those who have the qualifications.

1. A BORN TEACHER . . . Are you the type person who enjoys teaching someone else the things that you are capable of doing?
   - Do you derive pleasure from seeing someone progress . . . without fear of that person surpassing your own capabilities?
   - Can you take the responsibility for someone else's progress . . .?
     Are you aware that the TEACHER learns as much as the STUDENT learns when creative teaching is taking place?
   - When the student has difficulty learning, are you capable of finding NEW ways to say the same thing . . . understanding that the TEACHER and not the student is responsible for the learning process?

2. A "PEOPLE LOVER" . . . Working with various personalities day in and day out can be more than some people can handle. In order to teach successfully, the Teacher must genuinely enjoy PEOPLE. There are many dancers . . . artists . . . performers . . . gifted in their chosen field, but incapable of dealing with different personalities. One must have patience and a pride in the accomplishment of OTHERS in order to be a GOOD Teacher. There are thousands of Teachers. Many have become Teachers for all of the wrong reasons. Teaching should be regarded as a PRIVILEGE. The entrusting of the development and guidance of other human beings should not be taken lightly.

3. A TECHNICIAN . . . The dedicated Teacher of Dance in ANY form should be interested in the development of UP-TO-DATE teaching techniques and in constantly upgrading his own capabilities. Today is an ERA OF ACADEMIC EDUCATION. Students expect to be TAUGHT . . . not just SHOWN how to coordinate different parts of the body to varying tempos and styles. A knowledgeable Teacher should understand MORE than one specific area of Dance. The UNIVERSAL UNIT SYSTEM is a method of relating ALL FORMS of Dance to each other.

If YOU ARE CONSIDERING A CAREER OR AVOCATION TEACHING DANCE, consult your local DANCE INFORMATION BUREAU and make an appointment with a Counselor from the GOLDEN STATE DANCE TEACHERS ASSOCIATION. Many PERFORMERS . . . NATIONAL DANCE COMPETITION WINNERS . . . and hundreds of TEACHERS OF DANCE have been trained in the UNIVERSAL UNIT SYSTEM. Still the DEMAND far exceeds the SUPPLY for QUALIFIED TEACHERS . . . (PARTICULARLY in the CONTEMPORARY SOCIAL DANCE FIELD).

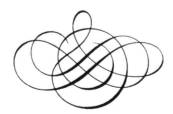

Golden State Dance Teachers Association

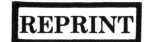

HOLISTIC APPROACH TO DANCE

Lecture—September 28, 1977

UNIVERSAL UNIT SYSTEM — the Holistic approach to dance. When one learns to read — all knowledge is his for the reading. When one learns to write . . . communication grows in leaps & bounds. When one learns to play a musical instrument he plays as in a Universal language through notes & scales that comprise all music. And when one learns the UNIVERSAL UNIT SYSTEM, the entire realm of DANCE is laid at his feet. Social Dance, Folk Dance, Creative Ballet, Jazz or even Contemporary Dances — a student of the UNIVERSAL UNIT SYSTEM will recognize & recreate that which he sees. There have been many innovative approaches to dance over the decades. Never before has one system so thoroughly accomplished an understanding of all areas of dance. A child schooled in the UNIVERSAL UNIT SYSTEM not only develops mind and body co-ordination unequal to any other training, but also learns musical interpretation, timing, phrasing, and all of the necessary elements to be comfortable & knowledgeable in any era of dance.

Social communication on a dance floor usually confines itself to the era in which the dancer attended school. Thus we are segregated by being Swing dancers — Balboa dancers — Twist dancers — Bugaloo dancers — Charleston dancers — each Era having their own clique. The average person confines his social dancing to the era in which he was the most popular . . . not by CHOICE or PREFERENCE but because that is the ONLY thing he knows. As dances are presented outside his era he does not understand them and is not able to produce them with a minimal amount of effort. The UNIVERSAL UNIT SYSTEM, with its holistic approach to dance, equips the individual with the basic knowledge of which all dance is composed. Never again need someone be embarrassed by not being able to participate when a new dance enters the social scene. Armed with the knowledge that all dance is equal to the sum total of its parts, a student of the UNIVERSAL UNIT SYSTEM can dissect those movements which he sees and relate those movements to the music which he hears. As incredible as it sounds, all the mystery has been taken out of learning how to dance.

Small children, given the opportunity to develop through the UNIVERSAL UNIT SYSTEM, do not have to go through what most people have referred to as the awkward stage. There need never be an awkward stage for those youngsters. When a child is small we teach him to talk and if he has a speech impediment we work to make his pronunciation clearer. We hire a tutor to see to it that his speech is acceptable in our society. If he cannot read, we get him a tutor so that he can keep up to the best of his ability. We teach him to eat with a knife & fork, . . . teach him table manners, . . . teach him how to tie his shoes, . . . and yet, if he puts one foot in front of the other and stands up-right, we assume that he knows how to walk. If he stumbles we assume he is a clumsy child. If he trips over things, we assume it is something he will outgrow and yet NO ONE TEACHES HIM the basic co-ordination that he needs in order to function properly. If a child is awkward or if an adult is awkward, people react to him as if he were less than an agile co-ordinated human being. And when someone reacts to us as if we are inferior there is something within us that reacts by BECOMING inferior. And so it is in all training that we try to co-ordinate both the mind and the body to develop each person to their highest potential.

The UNIVERSAL UNIT SYSTEM gives a person guidelines in rhythmic movement and co-ordination development. This training produces a look of confidence, agility & intelligence. Yes . . . there IS a look of intelligence on the face of that person who feels comfortable and confident in every situation. By helping develop these traits, we develop that thing within each individual that makes everyday living a joyous experience. That comes with the confidence that one can handle any situation. CONFIDENCE grows through series of successes. The UNIVERSAL UNIT SYSTEM creates a series of successes. . . . There are no failures. This series of guided movements, along with the visual aids that relate one to the other, has guidelines and work projects which chart the progress of the individual. The student can SEE his own progress.

Many teachers of dance have been amazed at the results of the UNIVERSAL UNIT SYSTEM. One particular fact has been outstanding. The very talented individual who has to work very little to keep time to music or move with co-ordination . . . that person who has inborn talent . . . who has NO difficulty in picking up material . . . it is that particular person, at the end of the course, who is not always the best dancer in the group. The holistic approach brings up that individual who was at the bottom of the heap and gives him a chance to be up there at the top. Diligence, patience, hard work is rewarded & the feeling of accomplishment in the teacher is something to be experienced. It is no great contribution to society to take a talented individual and show him something and have him do it well. That does not require teaching or method or much of anything but passing along information. The test of a true teacher of a teaching system is to take that individual who has difficulty with timing, co-ordination, movement, etc. and turn him into a graceful, co-ordinated, musically oriented individual. This is the crux of the system.

Golden State Dance Teachers Association

MEMO to TEACHERS OF THE UNIVERSAL UNIT SYSTEM, May 1978

In recent NEW Teacher Training Sessions, here are The THREE MOST FREQUENTLY ASKED QUESTIONS CONCERNING THE USE OF THE UNIVERSAL UNIT SYSTEM.

1. If a UNIT is defined as having only TWO BEATS OF MUSIC, how do we justify a SYNCOPATED TRIPLE which requires 2½ beats of music to complete?

Answer: In MUSIC, at an advanced stage, the musician inserts a "GRACE" note at the beginning of a measure because MUSICALLY it belongs with THAT PARTICULAR MEASURE. He has BORROWED that note from the previous measure. In the DANCE, at an advanced stage, we BORROW half a note from the previous UNIT in order to put the STEP where it belongs in relationship to the desired movement of the pattern being danced. The PATTERN is still done within the framework of a specific number of beats. It has not altered the number of beats of music . . . only the PLACEMENT for maximum creative expression.

2. Why do we use the term WALTZ MEASURE instead of having a WALTZ UNIT?

Answer: In MUSIC, we have taken a 4/4 time MEASURE and broken it in HALF to its smallest UNIT. (HALF a measure contains two equal UNITS, both of which contain a DOWNBEAT and an UPBEAT.) In WALTZ, which is 3/4 time, the MEASURE is complete in itself. It cannot be condensed or cut in half. It contains ONE DOWNBEAT and TWO UPBEATS. It is not a PART of something else.

3. How can I tell from the UNITS whether you are referring to the FREE FOOT or the WEIGHTED FOOT?

Answer: The SLASHES refer to the FREE FOOT. The DOTS refer to the WEIGHTED FOOT. OPEN CIRCLES are either HOPS or smaller movements of the SAME FOOT. Any SOLID DOT is a transfer of weight to the OTHER FOOT. Any SLASH, representing a KICK, a TOUCH, a BRUSH, a LIFT or WHATEVER . . . can only be done by the FREE FOOT (NO WEIGHT!!)

NOTE: The BASIC RHYTHM UNITS . . . the actual UNIT CARDS and their subsequent ADVANCED UNIS, etc. are merely the BEGINNING of an INTRODUCTION to the whole system. The UNIVERSAL UNIT SYSTEM is a complete system of RHYTHMS, MOVEMENT, COORDINATION TRAINING, CHOREOGRAPHY, CREATIVE DEVELOPMENT, LOGIC TRAINING, and a foundation for the underlying relationship of every dance form to each other.

To see the UNIVERSAL UNIT SYSTEM as a series of SINGLE DOUBLE and TRIPLE RHYTHM UNIT CARDS . . . is the same as learning to play the scale on the PIANO and assuming that PLAYING THE SCALE ON THE PIANO is the sum total of MUSIC. The SCALE becomes the SUM TOTAL of that individual's EXPERIENCE and KNOWLEDGE of music. As KNOWLEDGE GROWS, the experience of the nature of MUSIC grows. As your knowledge of the UNIVERSAL UNIT SYSTEM grows, your knowledge of the all encompassing form of DANCE will grow. There is NO PIECE OF MUSIC that cannot be written . . . and there is NO MOVEMENT done in time to music, that cannot be translated into the UNIT SYSTEM.

REVERSING that procedure, if one studies DANCE in the form laid out by the UNIVERSAL UNIT SYSTEM, he will understand ALL DANCE . . . ALL MOVEMENT . . . ALL RHYTHM . . . and better still, he will understand HIMSELF. To KNOW is to UNDERSTAND. The UNIVERSAL UNIT SYSTEM is a way toward UNDERSTANDING.

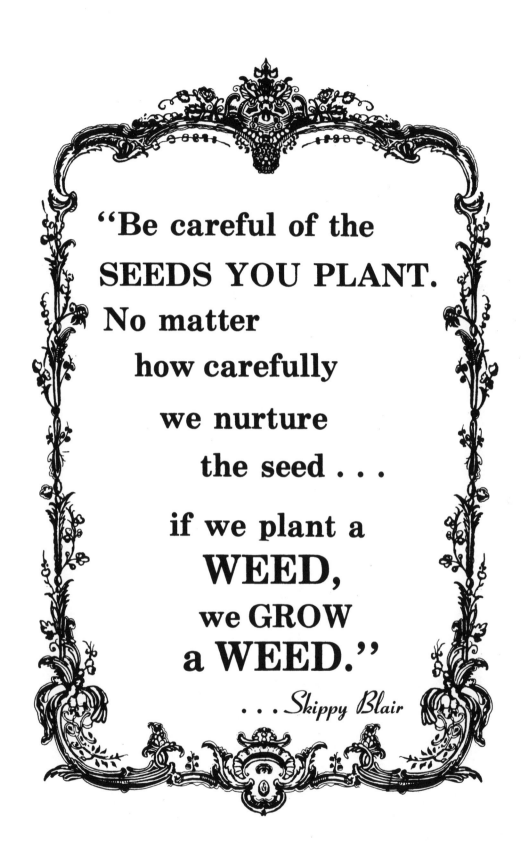

"Be careful of the
SEEDS YOU PLANT.
No matter
how carefully
we nurture
the seed . . .
if we plant a
WEED,
we GROW
a WEED."

. . . *Skippy Blair*

Chapter XII
CHILDREN AND THE UNIVERSAL UNIT SYSTEM

The UNIVERSAL UNIT SYSTEM is a system of teaching movement and dance. It also is a method of developing mind and body coordination. The U.U.S. has been accepted in many of the public and private schools and is being taught in several California Colleges.

The BENEFITS of this training are many. The younger the child, the easier is the acceptance of the knowledge. Armed with the knowledge that the system presents, a child need never go thru the "awkward stage." Students of the U.U.S. develop their coordination to a degree that assists them in ANY physical endeavor. They become better athletes, or dancers, or just more coordinated human beings.

In later years, the student is able to recognize (and duplicate) new dance forms that we have no way of predicting today. Thus, we are eliminating the wallflowers of tomorrow.

Included in this text are comments from Grade School teachers who participated in a Summer Program at Killian School. Also comments from the year round program at "Our Lady of Perpetual Help," Parochial School in Downey, California.

If you can visualize the brain as a computer, you will get a picture of how the Unit System works to coordinate the mind and body of a youngster. The IMPORTANT part is to see that we do not feed in any information that you do not wish to keep. By having the children learn their FOOT POSITIONS and the various RHYTHM UNITS, they learn to KEEP TIME TO MUSIC. They also learn the different relationships of EVEN and ODD numbers. (There have been many reports of increased interest in arithmetic. Some, not so much of INTEREST, but of better UNDERSTANDING.) A knowledge of the FOOT POSITIONS and quick CHANGES OF WEIGHT gives the child who has not been all that coordinated a chance to LEARN coordination, control . . . and BALANCE.

Why do we assume that because a child puts one foot in front of the other and does not fall down that he has LEARNED TO WALK? Many children develop bad habits that will lead to bad backs, headaches and all kinds of disorders later on in life. Being told to WALK STRAIGHT will not accomplish anything. However, learning that people who ARE SOMEBODY . . . Those who KNOW THEY ARE WORTHWHILE . . . walk with their heads up and their feet in FOURTH FOOT POSITION does amazing things to a school classroom. Try it yourself . . . Walk a TIGHTROPE (or a Balance Beam), pressing the top of your head toward the ceiling and moving across the floor as if you were really walking the rope. You will find that there is more oxygen moving into the lungs and a feeling of WELL BEING settles around you. Yes . . . part of the system of UNIT TRAINING includes HOW TO BREATHE. (See Chapter III.)

Golden State Dance Teachers Association

Reprint from DANCE VIEWS Publication, 1974

REPRINT

UNIVERSAL UNIT SYSTEM

. . . A PROGRESS REPORT . . . by SKIPPY BLAIR

. . . The SUMMER SCHOOL classes that BETTY SCHEULER taught at KILLIAN SCHOOL have now been evaluated. Some of the "Homeroom" teachers have written comments regarding the class. Excerpts follow: (Classes taught were Kindergarten thru Fifth Grade.)

. . . "children in my classes progressed noticeably: in movement to music in time with basic meter, in overall large muscle response, in use of their bodies for expression with unexpected poise, and in general listening ability" . . . CORA ASHBY

(Ms. Ashby has 10 years experience as a FIRST GRADE teacher and also states that she is convinced that the RHYTHM PROGRAM, if presented on a regular basis, would aid in the overall reading and general learning skills.)

. . . "My class had a minimum of instruction time but seem to have benefited noticeably. Most of them learned the difference between SINGLE RHYTHM and DOUBLE RHYTHM and could clap as well as march to the beats of the music . . . program would help develop more coordination in these younger children" . . . SANDY BILLODEAU

(Kindergarten Teacher at Killian School)

. . . ". . . aware of the direct correlation between large and small muscle coordination and academic achievement . . . program is an excellent one and very well structured, encouraging ALL children to participate at their own pace . . . CLAIRE SKAGGS (3rd & 4th grade teacher) . . . JOYCE FLACK (4th & 5th grade teacher)

The UNIVERSAL UNIT SYSTEM can be taught from Pre-school thru Senior Citizen level . . . and in each case, it will increase the mental and physical coordination of the individual. It is now being used as a learning tool in MUSIC and PHYSICAL EDUCATION as well as the dance. Any TEACHER of dance or ANYONE who takes his dancing seriously, owes it to himself to explore this new concept. It will AMAZE you!

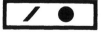 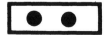 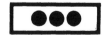

The following POEMS are for use with teaching young CHILDREN. Frequently, these little poems have been responsible for an ADULT being able to remember the three different Rhythms. The MUSIC is very important in learning RHYTHMS. Always pick out music that has an EVEN STEADY BEAT ... one that makes it easy to TAP YOUR FOOT in RHYTHM.

For teaching CHILDREN, the VISUAL ASPECT is even more important than the VERBAL. We suggest that you make LARGE UNIT CARDS, duplicating the UNITS that you see in this text. Cards can be purchased. However, white card stock and black construction paper can produce excellent VISUAL AIDS.

The DIMENSIONS of the UNIT CARDS are important. Many experiments have been conducted and the results have shown that our final UNIT CARD dimension is the most easily understood, read, and maintained.

UNIT CARD should be more than TWICE as LONG as it is HIGH. The DOTS should be HALF the height of the WHITE SPACE within the UNIT. The BORDER should be a heavy black line that sets it apart from whatever is behind it.

This dimension encourages the eye to travel from LEFT TO RIGHT, the same as we do in READING. Sheet music does the same thing ... travels the eye from Left to Right.

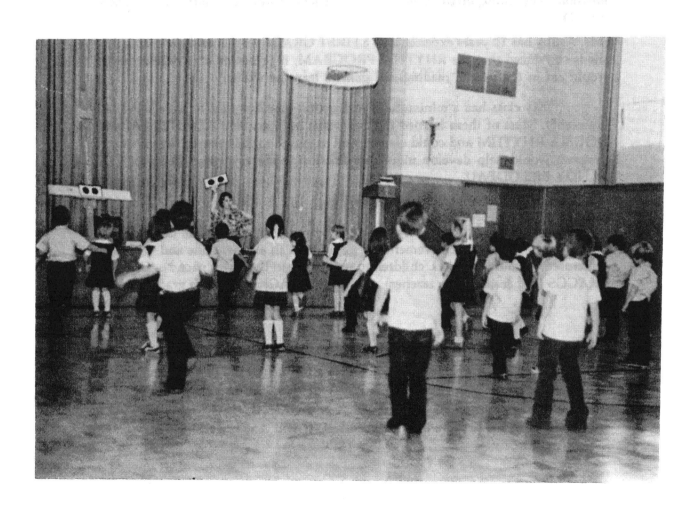

UNIT CARDS already made up are available from the Golden State Dance Teachers Association: 11120 Downey Ave., Downey, Calif. 90241.

CHILDREN'S UNIT SONGS ©1974

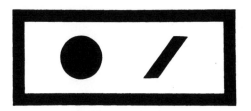

- I AM "SINGLE RHYTHM"
  'CAUSE I ONLY STEP ONE TIME . . .
I DO "STEP TOUCH . . . STEP TOUCH"
  AND SAY THIS LITTLE RHYME.

(. . . or Teacher can substitute "STEP KICK" or "STEP LIFT"
or whatever is being taught that day.)

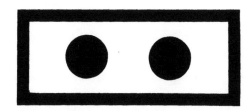

- I AM "DOUBLE RHYTHM." I GO MARCHING DOWN THE STREET.
  "LEFT RIGHT . . . LEFT RIGHT" . . . STEP ON EVERY BEAT.

(. . . then use "RIGHT LEFT . . . RIGHT LEFT")

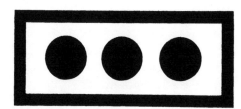

- I AM "TRIPLE RHYTHM."
  I AM FASTER THAN THE REST.
I GO "LEFT RIGHT LEFT and RIGHT LEFT RIGHT"
  WHEN I AM AT MY BEST.

THE O.L.P.H. "EXPERIENCE"

Sept. 17, 1978

by Skippy Blair

It was our first opportunity to see the UNIVERSAL UNIT SYSTEM in action for a full school year. Our Lady of Perpetual Help Parochial School in Downey, California had contracted for ONE HOUR a week for EACH GRADE LEVEL, Kindergarten thru Eighth Grade. This was to be the "follow up" to all of the summer and part-time experimental classes. It was . . . and it was great. Examinations at the conclusion of the school year showed a great deal more than just the learning of a few dance steps.

In the examination, several of the classes were asked: "If I know that I am a worthwhile individual and I REALLY AM somebody, I will walk in which FOOT POSITION?" Almost everyone of the youngsters answered FOURTH FOOT POSITION. (How good it is to walk down the hall and watch these young people AWARE of their carriage and standing tall.) Twice during the school year, we presented a program for the parents so that they could see the progress. The 6th, 7th and 8th grade students were able to perform some of the contemporary COUPLES DANCES (Slow dancing, Latin Hustle) and also the LINE HUSTLE as a group. The earlier grades danced various versions of the LINE HUSTLE, the SUNDANCE HUSTLE and the GET UP GET DOWN HUSTLE. The UNITS were much in evidence as each class performed their particular segment of the evening's entertainment.

Sister Mary Immaculette commented on the physical coordination training that the system provided. She was actually more "tickled" over the performance of the BASKETBALL TEAM than of the actual dancing itself. She said that they had lost their TALL players from the year before and the team was about 12th in the league. After all the UNIT TRAINING, their fast footwork carried them to FOURTH place in the league. She was very proud of the team. She was also very proud of the dancing itself. She had a right to be. These young people not only danced quite a few dance variations, but had learned the COMPONENTS that make up all dance. In the classes they were able to compose their own DANCE PATTERNS.

As DANCE EDUCATORS, we are more interested in the overall development of human potential . . . than in the mere execution of a few dance steps. However, in the process of teaching this physical and mental coordination with the UNIT SYSTEM . . . isn't the "BY PRODUCT" a fascinating one? These young people will be able to "see" the dances as they come up in the future . . . and DUPLICATE them . . . because they will recognize the UNITS of which they are composed.

One of the teachers reported a new "awareness" of simple mathematical problems by a student who had formerly been doing poorly in Arithmetic. The student became aware of the TWO BEAT UNIT and was able to add any EVEN numbers as if they were UNITS and could add any other set of numbers by seeing them as DOTS (steps). The concept is not a new one, but it certainly is rewarding to see the EXTRA benefits of the SYSTEM in ACTION.

The teachers for the first year at O.L.P.H. were Bette Mehlbrech and Gazel Valenzuela . . . two highly competent young ladies who are both CREDENTIALED SCHOOL TEACHERS with the State of California . . . as well as being trained, tested and approved by the Golden State Dance Teachers' Association in the UNIVERSAL UNIT SYSTEM.

The dance program at our school has elicited the most favorable comments I have ever heard from our parents. All Skippy has said above is true and more. Some of the greatest advantages I believe are creating self-confidence in the children, making them more socially acceptable, increasing motor coordination which is reflected in their school work as well as in their athletic ability, and making them a more well-rounded person. Another very important aspect of the program is that it provides discipline of mind and body.

In our school philosophy we state that we provide an education which includes the development of the whole child. I believe that the dance program is one that provides psychological, aesthetical and physical development and helps to improve spiritual and intellectual growth as well.

Since another of our basic goals is to provide a favorable climax where growth in faith through community is more readily achieved we believe that the dance program challenges the children to accept one another in the spirit of friendship and appreciation. We hope that through the skills the children have gained they may always be more acceptable in groups where the social graces enhance their lives and bring pleasure to others.

Sister Mary Immaculette
Sept. 22, 1978

P.S. I have enclosed a list of selected comments from the questionnaires that were returned to us.

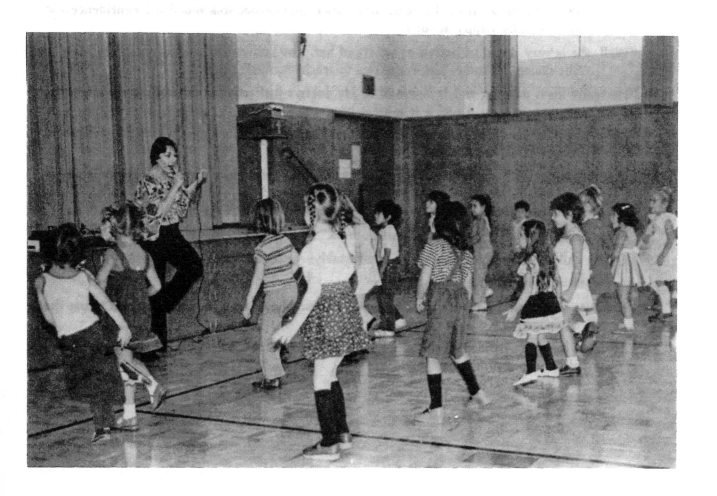

Parents Comments Concerning Dance Program:

- "They have become more involved with other children and are no longer shy."
- "They love to dance."
- "It has improved her coordination."
- "My child has developed a greater self-confidence."
- "Our daughter feels she is contributing something useful when the class can put on a performance. It is also another activity to look forward to."
- "He has more confidence in himself socially. I feel it has been most advantageous to him. I only wish my other two boys would have had the same opportunity."
- "My child developed more coordination and loves dancing."
- "She loves music and dancing because she really thinks she is expressing her feelings when she does this."
- "Brought my 8th grader out of a shell and my first grader is much more coordinated."
- "He enjoys music more and is not afraid to express himself."
- "More graceful; stimulates the brain."
- "Gives a sense of social success; can do the latest dances."
- "He really appreciates music and likes to watch adults dance and sing."
- "They feel important because they can dance now."
- "My daughter has always been awkward and I have noticed she feels so good about herself when she shows us what she has learned in dance. She needed this added self-confidence and we are really happy about it."
- "Well, she is very proud of herself as we are of her. She knows the latest dances. She loves it. She dances at home. She even tries to teach her little sister."
- "He really loves dancing and is aware of it. He doesn't just move around aimlessly when the music comes on. I feel it is a great program."
- "I hope there'll be more, because it has helped to make my child more coordinated physically and come out of her shyness."
- "Our 6th grader really enjoys it — the intricacies of some of the dance patterns really increase her coordination. Our 4th grader isn't too impressed yet but any involvement he experiences in the class is certainly better than nothing."
- "Poise, friendly activity and contact with others."
- "Oldest child was taught to mix more comfortably; youngest child loves it."
- "A greater rapport with others."
- "He loves music and he is well coordinated in sports. The dance class will help him to use the two together."
- "My girls are really thrilled with the program. It has also contributed to their imagination and after-school programs."

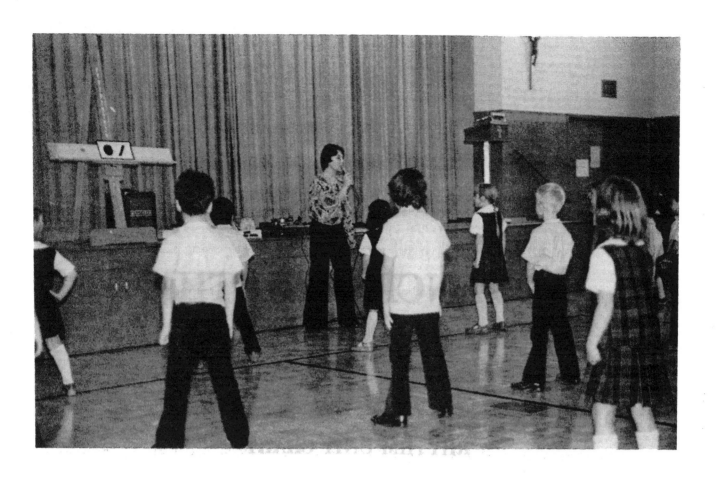

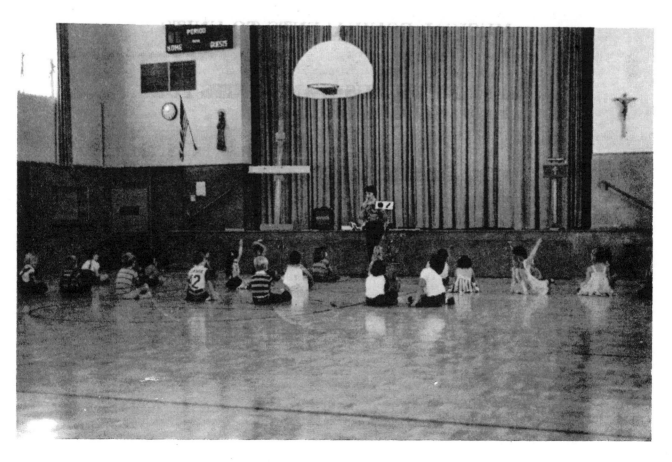

163

Chapter XIII

ADVANCED RHYTHM UNITS

RHYTHM UNIT CHART

MUSICAL EQUIVALENTS TO UNITS

REPRINT OF MUSIC AND UNITS FOR
SCHOOL CHILDREN

BASIC ANNOTATION

UNDERSTANDING THE RHYTHM UNIT CHART

On The Next Page You Will See The RHYTHM UNIT CHART, showing many variations of Single Rhythm, Double Rhythm, Triple Rhythm and even Blank Rhythm Units. When you STUDY the first column of the SINGLE RHYTHM chart, you will not only see four different versions of Single Rhythm, but you will see how they are discovered. YOU will be able to work out all the different Rhythms, even if you do not have the chart with you.

Look at the first one. The ONE DOT is "far left", on the first "&" count. It is a "Syncopated Single". The one under that is a regular SINGLE RHYTHM UNIT with the ONE DOT under count "1". The next DOT is on the "&" after the "1" and is another "Syncopated Single". The fourth Unit places the DOT on count "2", which is a Delayed Single. Notice that in each consecutive unit the DOT moves over one space. This produces a different kind of "Single Rhythm" with each move.

The discovery of this process of finding the various RHYTHM UNITS makes it possible for you to know every rhythm that has ever been danced and every rhythm that ever WILL be danced. COUNT THE DOTS. Those ARE the weight changes.

Take ANY Pattern in ANY DANCE (Ballroom, Country, Latin, International, Swing, Jazz, Ballet etc.) and pick out your most complicated syncopation (any two beat rhythm). Chances are, you will find the Unit is already on the Unit Chart. If not, you have the formula for making the Unit yourself. Being able to separate each Rhythm Unit, in each pattern, gives you a different view of the pattern itself...and expands your overall knowledge of the dance.

In identifying SYNCOPATIONS we step on the "&" counts and sometimes do something else (Kick, Lift, Touch, etc.) on the actual beat of music. In the Rhythm Unit, Slashes are always placed on the Beat of Music, if no weight change takes place on that count.

Rhythm Units are broken into 4 parts (see schematic) and those time values are counted "&1&2". However, at a more advanced level of syncopated movement, we find that the "time value" changes for the "&" counts. A "rolling triple", as found in West Coast Swing or in Samba, shares the time space of the "&" count and becomes "&a". Thus, the more advanced Rhythm Unit uses 6 time values and is counted "&a1&a2". (see schematic) This count is invaluable for breaking down more complicated internal movement flow.

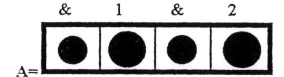

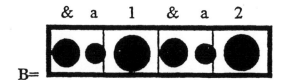

RHYTHM UNIT CHART

For Unlimited Rhythm Variations, substitute any "ODD" RHYTHM UNIT for any other "ODD" Rhythm Unit.....or any "EVEN" RHYTHM UNIT for any other "EVEN" RHYTHM UNIT

(2 BEAT UNIT = 1 DOWN Beat and 1 UP Beat)

SINGLE RHYTHM UNITS   BLANK RHYTHM UNITS

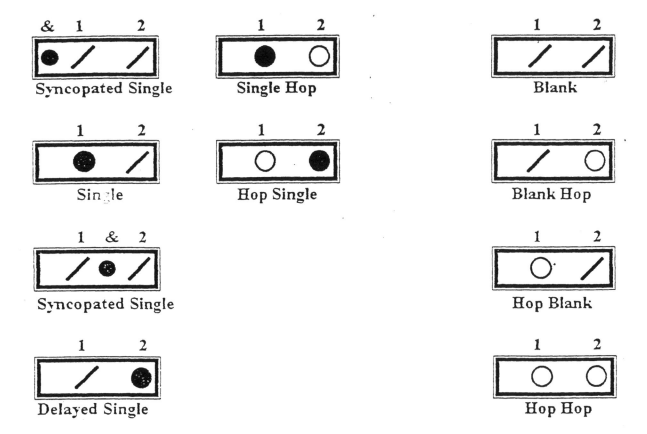

DOUBLE RHYTHM UNITS

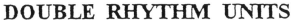

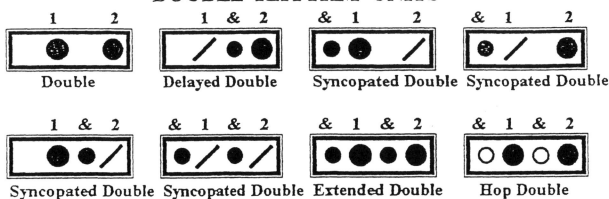

TRIPLE RHYTHM UNITS

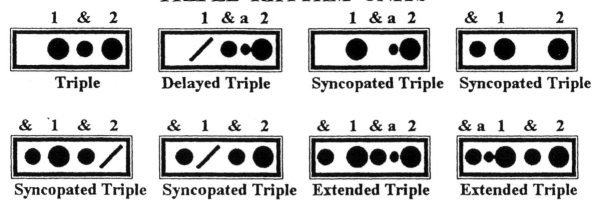

1 & 2	1 & a 2	1 & a 2	& 1 2
Triple	Delayed Triple	Syncopated Triple	Syncopated Triple

& 1 & 2	& 1 & 2	& 1 & a 2	& a 1 & 2
Syncopated Triple	Syncopated Triple	Extended Triple	Extended Triple

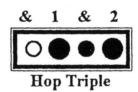

& 1 & 2

Hop Triple

3 BEAT UNITS

(3 BEAT UNIT = 1 DOWN Beat and 2 UP Beats)

Danced to 3/4 Time (Waltz)

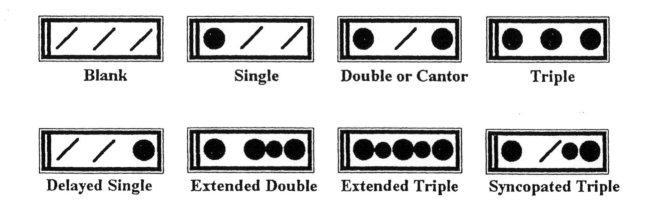

Blank	Single	Double or Cantor	Triple
Delayed Single	Extended Double	Extended Triple	Syncopated Triple

RELATING THE "RHYTHM UNITS"
TO SHEET MUSIC
(For those with a little or a lot of musical knowledge)

Relating The DANCE to the MUSIC is really what learning to dance is all about. If dancing was exactly like playing a musical instrument, we could dance to sheet music and there would be no need for Rhythm Units. Sheet music (in 4/4 time) is written in MEASURES of music. That MEASURE is four beats of music. There are so many things that a dancer could do in four beats of music that it would be impossible to list or categorize.

Dancers actually dance to "Two Beat" increments, composed of one DOWN-BEAT and one UP-BEAT. There are relatively few "Two Beat" increments in the DANCE.(see RHYTHM CHART on pages 166 & 167) The discovery of "THE SYSTEM" brought with it, the need for dancing to those Two Beat increments, and the REASONS why they must be recognized. .

In MUSIC, little extra notes ("&a") follow AFTER a beat of music.. A musician could count a measure as "1 e & a" - "2 e & a" - "3 e & a" - "4 e & a". In DANCE, we not only confine the RHYTHMS to two beats of music, we also "syncopate" our rhythms BEFORE the count. In music, that would be similar to playing a "pick up" note or a "grace" note.

Many Syncopations are danced with "pick up" rhythms. Here are a few of the more recognizable SYNCOPATIONS that use the "&" before the beat:

"& 1 2" could be "Step Kick Step" or "Step Step Hold" or " Step Step Step"
"& 1 & 2" could be "Step Point Step Point" or "Step Kick Step Point"
"& 1 & a 2" could be "Step Kick Step Step Step" or "Step Step HOLD Step Step"

The discovery of the RHYTHM UNIT is as important to a dancer as sheet music is to a musician. There is no piece of music that can be played on a piano that cannot be translated to sheet music. Some music is more DIFFICULT to translate, but an accomplished musician can do it. There are complicated moves in dance that require advanced knowledge of rhythm units, but there are NO dance moves (that fit to music) that cannot be translated into RHYTHM UNITS .

Please do not relate the DOTS to quarter notes. They are WEIGHT CHANGES (generally STEPS). The COUNT tells you where those weight changes take place. The SIZE of the DOTS will help to identify the count. The LARGE Dot is on the actual Beat of music. The MEDIUM sized Dot is an "&" count and the SMALL Dot is an "a" count.

The next page shows some "note" values that should answer questions for musicians. For further clarification, contact the GOLDEN STATE DANCE TEACHERS ASSOCIATION, a National, non-profit organization with headquarters in Downey, California. (see inside cover)

Relationship of Units to: SHEET MUSIC

FOR THE MUSIC STUDENT:
A few comparisons of note values.

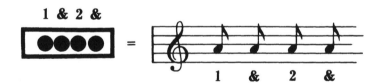

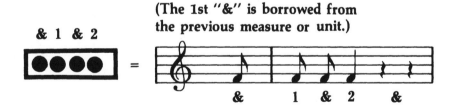

(The 1st "&" is borrowed from the previous measure or unit.)

(1st "&" borrowed from previous unit.)

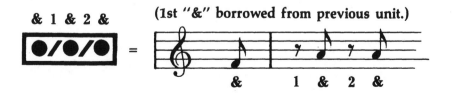

Rhythm dances "breathe," "turn," or "lift" between the units.

Smooth dances flow thru the units (Body Flight) but still maintain the timing of the individual units.

Basic Annotation for the UNIVERSAL UNIT SYSTEM

In this book, covering the concept of the UNIVERSAL UNIT SYSTEM, the emphasis has been placed on LEARNING HOW TO DANCE. In many of the chapters the annotation changes from time to time to gently guide the mind toward the total annotation system itself. A complete breakdown on annotation would be a whole new book. In this one, we are including the basic form which will be helpful in writing down material in an understandable "shorthand" form.

F = Forward (4th foot position)

B = Back (4th foot position)

S = Left or Right in the direction of the FREE FOOT. (2nd foot position)

T = Together, heels touching, toes SLIGHTLY apart (1st foot position)

X = One foot stepping OVER the other (in front) . . . a CROSS

Hk = a HOOK where the free foot hooks behind the weighted foot before stepping.

( ) = No weight change. In the parenthesis any of the above symbols can be used to designate DIRECTION of the free foot

(K) = Kick $\langle$ =Conversation position=Both partners facing same direction on an angle.

CW = Clockwise   Hp=Hop

CCW = Counter Clockwise

▲___ = the direction of the man's C.P.B. in relationship to a forward wall or to his partner.

△___ = the direction of the girl's C.P.B. in relationship to a forward wall or to her partner.

▷ ···· ◁ = partners facing each other, his LEFT hand to her RIGHT hand.

▲ △ = partners "side by side"

If further explanation is needed for hand postion, the use of a straight solid line indicates the RIGHT ARM. (not always used.)

A broken line, or little dashes, indicates the LEFT ARM.

Arrows placed between units indicate a TURN in the direction of the arrow. If the arrow is AROUND the DOT, the turn takes place ON the COUNT.

Arrows indicate the direction of a turn. . .or a kick. . .or a hand move. If the arrow is between the units, the turn is on the & between the units. If the arrow is around the DOT, the turn takes place ON THE COUNT.

COMPARISON OF UNITS TO WORDS . . .

A-B-Cs=BEATS OF MUSIC

WORDS=UNITS

SENTENCES=PATTERNS (SCHOOL FIGURES)

PARAGRAPHS=AMALGAMATIONS (GROUP OF PATTERNS)
          MINOR OR MAJOR PHRASES

STORY=COMPLETE ROUTINE:
- OPENING
- MANY "PARAGRAPHS"
- HIGHLIGHT (ONE OR SEVERAL)
- ENDING

Musically, most of the SYNCOPATIONS are a splitting up of the first quarter note
. . . or the first beat.

• SAMBA TRIPLE . . . count: 1 & a 2. The "2" is a full beat. The "1 & a" is a beat that has been broken up into a dotted eighth note and a sixteenth note.

• TWO STEP TRIPLE . . . equals two eighth notes for "1 &" and a quarter note for "2."

• A Syncopated DOUBLE "borrows" an eighth note from the previous unit. The count is: "& 1 & 2." The "& 1 &" are all eighth notes, followed by a quarter note for "2."

• A Syncopated TRIPLE also borrows the eighth note from the previous unit. The count is: "& 1 & 2 &." Each count would be an eighth note. The 1st "&" is the one that is borrowed. The rest (4 eighth notes) equal the 2 quarter notes of the Unit.

MUSIC:

• 1 MEASURE 4/4 TIME=4 BEATS=2 UNITS
• ½ MEASURE 4/4 TIME=2 BEATS=1 UNIT

• 1 MEASURE 3/4 TIME=3 BEATS=1 WALTZ MEASURE:

• DOWN-BEAT . . . The downbeat refers to the 1st and 3rd beats of music in a measure of 4/4 time. There are four "quarter notes" to a measure in almost all rhythm dances. (Some Sambas are written in 2/4.) The drummer may ACCENT EITHER the downbeat OR the upbeat, but their LOCATION will be the same! Many of the Latin rhythms accent the upbeat . . . also much of the jazz music accents the upbeat . . . It was a natural turn of events when jazz and Latin drummers played dance music . . . the result was Rock & Roll . . . (and all of its descendants!) For years the American dancing public had been accustomed to accenting the downbeat. Little wonder that adults did not understand the "younger generation" when they first observed them doing Rock & Roll.

• UP-BEAT . . . The 2nd and 4th beats of music in 4/4 time are the upbeat. Accenting the upbeat produces interesting variations of many of the rhythm dances!! Every "UNIT" consists of one downbeat and one upbeat!!

• INVERTED UNIT . . . for easier understanding of the LATIN RHYTHMS, the unit STARTS on the UPBEAT. One measure: 2 3 . . . 4 & 5 . . . 6 7 . . . 8 & 1.

The Use of the "AND" COUNT for TEACHING PURPOSES and ANNOTATION

In practicing the individual UNITS it is a good idea to actually LIFT the foot on "AND" between the UNITS. Practicing SINGLE RHYTHM, count ONE TWO. . .AND. . .THREE FOUR. The RULE OF THE "AND" COUNT is this:

The "AND" between the UNITS can be a MOVEMENT (turn). . .or a LIFTING OF THE FOOT, ready for placement in the next UNIT. . .or just a breathing space to separate the Units. However. . .as soon as we STEP on that "AND" count, we must place it WITHIN one of the UNITS. The decision as to where it is placed is an easy one. If we are replacing BASIC UNITS with SYNCOPATIONS, we would place the "AND" count in the UNIT that is being replaced.

Example: If we replace the ANCHOR TRIPLE in SWING, (the last UNIT in a pattern) we are replacing the last UNIT. The syncopation would belong IN THAT UNIT.

5 and 6 would become and 5 and 6 and

In this instance, we are keeping all of the steps in the UNIT THAT IS BEING REPLACED. Could that FIRST "AND" COUNT be moved into the previous Unit? Yes it could. . .if it served any particular purpose. However, in this instance it is expedient to REPLACE a BASIC TRIPLE with a SYNCOPATED TRIPLE and therefore only have to change ONE UNIT instead of TWO. (see Syncopated Units.)

Try to think of that "AND" count as FLEXIBLE. . .NOT in its placement in the MUSIC. That remains the same. But FLEXIBLE in that it can be placed in one of THREE places.

1. BETWEEN the UNITS (as a BREATH to LIFT the foot, or TURN etc.)

2. At the END of a UNIT after the SECOND COUNT of the Unit. (This is comparable to breaking up the quarter note into eights.)

3. At the BEGINNING of a Unit if it belongs with the MOVEMENT of that Unit. . .or if it is necessary for the UNIT that is being replaced. (In this instance the "AND" is borrowed from the PREVIOUS UNIT which CANNOT use an "AND" count in the same spot.

4. Deduction. . . .There can only be ONE "AND" between any two counts. The choreographer has the choice of WHERE to place it to achieve the desired result.

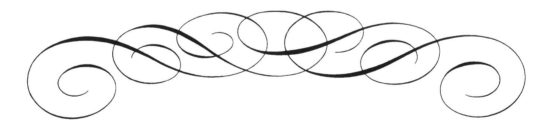

𝕲𝖔𝖑𝖉𝖊𝖓 𝕾𝖙𝖆𝖙𝖊 𝕯𝖆𝖓𝖈𝖊 𝕿𝖊𝖆𝖈𝖍𝖊𝖗𝖘 𝕬𝖘𝖘𝖔𝖈𝖎𝖆𝖙𝖎𝖔𝖓

RELATIONSHIP TO MUSIC   ⟦REPRINT⟧

Golden State Dance Teachers Association, April 8, 1975

To relate the UNIVERSAL UNIT SYSTEM to MUSIC as well as the dance, the following is of special interest.

1. Students of music, many of whom play an instrument fairly well, have had consistently bad scores on basic dance exams in TIMING! This problem has been reported in grade levels I thru Professional level over the past 20 years.

2. Students who have enrolled in UNIT CLASSES improve their TIMING and understanding of the RHYTHM VARIATIONS in less than ten hours (Class time).

3. In control study groups, we placed ten students with one teacher and ten with another . . . one using the UNIT SYSTEM, the other using standard teaching procedures. BOTH groups kept time to music while the class was in progress . . . and both SEEMED to understand the same things. However, separated from the teacher, the UNIT SYSTEM group maintained their timing and understanding. The other group was AVERAGE in the percentage that maintained both (30%).

4. The experiment was repeated reversing the teachers so that the personal proficiency of the teacher did not influence the results. The results were the same.

5. Students of dance who have reached a level of competition style dancing and STILL cannot phrase or even keep accurate timing have always been considered "non-dancers" . . . a phrase reserved for those who LEARN how to dance, but are never quite "with it." We have been able to teach these people how to STAY in time . . . how to PHRASE . . . and even how to choreograph their own material. The CREATIVE ELEMENT is the one that fascinates me most.

6. The MOVEMENT EXERCISES that are connected with the UNIVERSAL UNIT SYSTEM are quite similar to those being used to work with "hard to teach" youngsters in order to improve their reading readiness.

7. In direct proportion to the amount of UNIT STUDY, we have case after case of improved POSTURE . . . improved COORDINATION . . . improved BASIC PHYSICAL SKILLS . . . and a tremendous improvement in the INTEREST in MUSIC as well as the dance.

A UNIT deals with only TWO BEATS OF MUSIC. (A MEASURE covers too much ground.)

One DOT represents one WEIGHT CHANGE (in dance) or one CLAP in music appreciation.

Students learn to relate a SERIES of UNITS to any music they hear. A "/" represents a beat of music, but NO weight change (no CLAP) . . . the same as a "REST." We are dealing here with QUARTER NOTES (as if the music was 4/4 time). It is a very simple matter to GRADUATE to measures and half notes etc., once the student REALLY understands the BASIC RHYTHMS. We refer to these BASIC RHYTHMS as:

> SINGLE RHYTHM . . . ONE DOT to two beats of music
>
> DOUBLE RHYTHM . . . TWO DOTS to two beats of music
>
> TRIPLE RHYTHM . . . THREE DOTS to two beats of music

Armed with this knowledge, the student can learn all kinds of variations of rhythms. It becomes invaluable in the dance . . . because ALL SOCIAL DANCE (including "Folk," "Square," "Rock," etc.) is composed of these SAME BASIC UNITS and their extensions. A student learns to READ what he sees in the dance. He learns to HEAR and identify RHYTHM CHANGES in music.

Prepared for Whittier School District P.T.A. to show the relationship of Unit Training to Music.

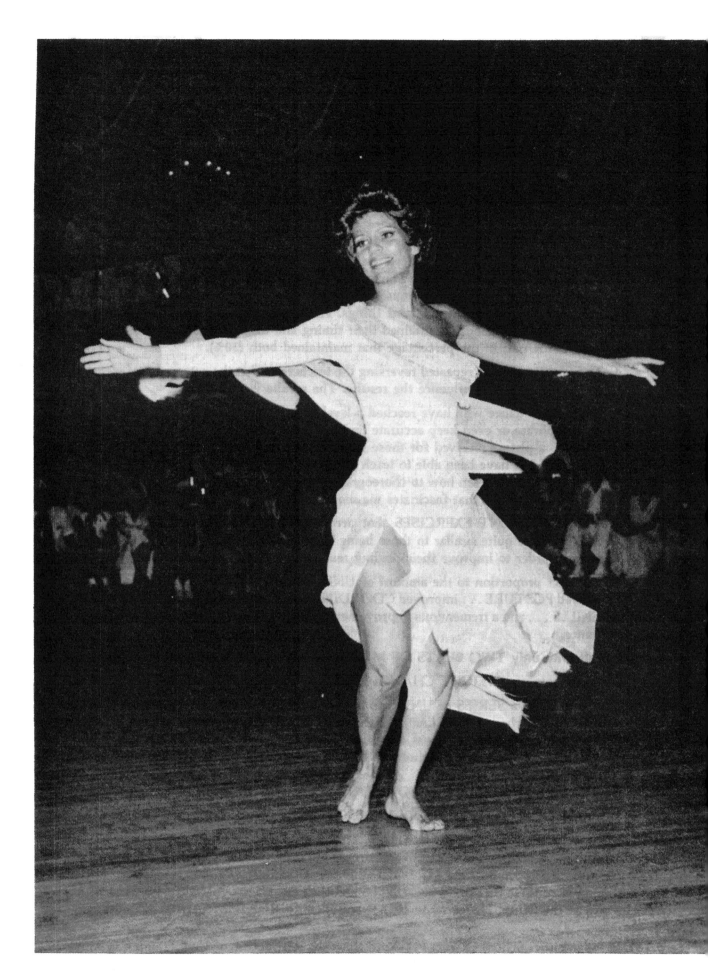

Chapter XIV
TERMINOLOGY

Terminology as it relates to the UNIVERSAL UNIT SYSTEM. We are aware that there are broader definitions for some of the terms used here. The definitions included here are for CLARIFICATION OF THE TERMS USED for the UNIVERSAL UNIT SYSTEM Method of DANCE TRAINING and ANNOTATION.

ACCENT . . . Emphasis on a particular count of music . . . or on a particular move in a Dance Pattern. The most widely used ACCENT is on the first beat of a measure.

ADVANCED RHYTHM UNITS . . . Refers to the 3rd stage of RHYTHM UNIT TRAINING. Those Units that are more complicated than the Primary and Secondary Units are the advanced SYNCOPATIONS (also includes a DELAYED TRIPLE).

AMALGAMATION . . . The joining of a series of patterns to form an interesting grouping. Good teaching, and therefore good Dancing should include amalgamations that phrase to the music.

ANCHOR UNIT . . . Refers to the last Unit of Golden State or California SWING. The "ANCHOR" refers to that feeling of body leverage that gives the man the control he needs to begin the next pattern.

"AND" . . . In the Universal UNIT SYSTEM the use of the "AND" count is most important. It is the BREATH between the UNITS. It is the movement that adds character to the dance. It is the pulse of the dance. (See explanation "Use of the "AND" count" in Chapter FOR TEACHERS ONLY.)

ASSIMILATION PERIOD . . . Refers to the time it takes to absorb that which is taught. In teaching Dance Classes it is advisable to have a 5 or 1 minute ASSIMILATION PERIOD at the end of every hour. (For taking notes, asking questions, or just for a supervised practice period.)

BALL CHANGE . . . A TAP DANCING term, included here because of common usage. Not used in the UNIVERSAL UNIT SYSTEM except in TAP or MODERN JAZZ. The use of "BALL CHANGE" as a "CALL" sometimes produces movement inappropiate to the dance being done.

BASIC RHYTHM . . . The fundamental Rhythm of a particular Dance. For example: In FOX-TROT, Basic Rhythm is considered to be a SINGLE, SINGLE, DOUBLE . . . or a "SLOW, SLOW, QUICK QUICK."

BEAT . . . Refers to ONE BEAT OF MUSIC (a QUARTER NOTE).

BREAK . . . A change of direction, as in CHA CHA or MAMBO. (See also RHYTHM BREAKS.)

BODY FLIGHT . . . That indefinable feeling of "ONENESS" in movement that connects one dancer with the other in a cooperative flow to the music. The LEVERAGE that is visible as TWO people moving as ONE . . . either in the same direction . . . or as individuals on an elastic band that has one common center point.

BOUNCE . . . A "DOWN DOWN" movement, like a bouncing ball. A rhythmic lilt of the body achieved by relaxing the knees on the actual beat of the music. SAMBA is considered to have a MOVEMENT UNIT of a SUBTLE BOUNCE. (Subtle meaning that the bounce is felt but not seen.)

CALIFORNIA SHUFFLE . . . A type of SWING that uses all advanced syncopations and extends 6 beat patterns into 8 beats by continuing the syncopation (popular 1978).

CALIFORNIA SWING . . . Another name for WESTERN or WEST COAST SWING, except that the styling is considered more UP, with more Contemporary flavor.

CALL . . . The "CALL" is the COMMAND or VERBAL PATTERN that precedes the step to be done. In the UNIVERSAL UNIT SYSTEM it is suggested that the CALL for the next pattern be verbalized on the last Unit of the previous pattern.

CAMEL HIP . . . A projection of the HIP to the SAME SIDE as the WEIGHTED FOOT. For instance: If the FOOT UNIT steps LEFT RIGHT, the Hip will move to the same side, LEFT RIGHT. (See also Cuban Hip for contrast.)

CENTER POINT OF BALANCE . . . (abbreviated C.P.B.) The SOLAR PLEXUS. The Center from which all movement projects. (See Chapter on MOVEMENT.)

C.B.M. . . . (See Contra Body Movement.)

CHA CHA . . . A FOUR UNIT PATTERN Dance, composed of DOUBLE, TRIPLE, DOUBLE, TRIPLE in its Basic form. Cha Cha is an outgrowth of Mambo. Part of the Latin Family of Dances, the Cha Cha was once considered a "Fad" Dance, but now has become one of the American STANDARDS.

CHARLESTON . . . One of the All-time favorites as an American Classic, The Charleston was also considered a shocking Dance in its time. Basic Charleston is all SINGLE RHYTHM. (See Chapter on FAD DANCES.)

CHASSE' . . . (Pronounced Shah-say) A "Side Together" . . . Two beats of music stepping on each beat, 2nd Foot position to First Foot position . . . DOUBLE RHYTHM.

CHOREOGRAPHER . . . One who puts together routines to fit a specific piece of music. (One can also Choreograph without music to a specific time span.)

CHOREOGRAPHY . . . Refers to Routines or groups of moves and patterns planned in a way that someone can repeat them at a future time. The WORKS of a Choreographer.

CLASSIC DANCE . . . Ballet is considered the Classic Dance Form. However, in Dance Terminology for SOCIAL DANCE, we refer to the CLASSICS as those Dances which have become STANDARDS. When a specific Dance has become an ART FORM, we consider it a CLASSIC.

CONTEMPORARY SOCIAL DANCE . . . Refers to those Dances which are CURRENTLY in favor by the general public . . . and most particularly the COUPLE HUSTLE DANCES that are a product of the late 70's. (Latin Hustle, New York Hustle, Salsa etc.)

CONTRA BODY MOVEMENT . . . Left foot FORWARD while the Left shoulder is BACK . . . an exaggeration of a normal walking position.

C.P.B. . . . see Center Point of Balance.

CUBAN HIP . . . A projection of the HIP to the OPPOSITE SIDE from the WEIGHTED FOOT. For instance: If one steps LEFT RIGHT, the HIP would project RIGHT LEFT. (See Chapter on RUMBA.)

COUNT ... The actual BEATS OF MUSIC in a specific Pattern ... or Sets of EIGHT COUNTS for a Line Dance or Modern Jazz Routine. The important part of being able to COUNT is to be able to count ACTUAL BEATS of music and not FOOT PLACEMENTS. For instance: a TRIPLE is counted "ONE AND TWO" because it is only TWO BEATS OF MUSIC. To count the STEPS would train the ear to disregard the musical timing. (See Chapter on MUSIC and also COMPETITION.)

DANCE POSITION ... The position of One Partner in relationship to the other Partner (Two-Hand position, Closed, Solo, etc.).

DANCING VOCABULARY ... refers to those patterns and moves which a Dancer has committed to memory ... those patterns which are danced without special thought.

DELAYED RHYTHM UNITS ... There are THREE Delayed Rhythm Units (Delayed SINGLE, Delayed DOUBLE and Delayed TRIPLE). The "DELAY" refers to the fact that there is NO STEP on Count ONE of the Unit ... and yet the remainder of the steps are completed by Count TWO ([tap] STEP ... [kick] STEP STEP ... [kick] STEP STEP STEP).

DISCO DANCING ... The term "Disco" has been shortened from Discotheque, which referred to a PLACE where people danced to RECORDS instead of live music. Over a seven year period, the term DISCO has now come to mean a LOOK ... a SOUND ... a FEELING. The current (1978) DISCO DANCING refers to the current COUPLES DANCING including all of the various Hustles: Latin Hustle, New York Hustle, Newporter Salsa, Two Step, etc. DISCO MUSIC refers to Danceable Contemporary Music.

DISCO SWING ... (See SALSA and also read the "ESSENCE of CONTEMPORARY DANCE.")

D.J. ... The shortened version for "Disc Jockey," the person playing the records. Today the accomplished "Dee Jay" is an artist in his own right, blending one record into another without having to stop the music ... or the dancing.

DOT ... In the UNIVERSAL UNIT SYSTEM a SOLID DOT refers to a WEIGHT CHANGE (a STEP).

DOWN BEAT ... The 1st beat of a UNIT. ... The 1st and 3rd beat of a 4/4 time MEASURE. The 1st beat of a Waltz Measure. (Every UNIT is composed of one DOWNBEAT & one UPBEAT. Every WALTZ MEASURE is composed of one DOWNBEAT and two UPBEATS.)

DOUBLE RHYTHM ... Stepping two times to two beats of music ... Stepping on every beat, as in Marching. Double Rhythm starts with one foot free, and ends with the SAME foot free. It is an EVEN RHYTHM UNIT.

DRIVE ... The FORWARD or SIDEWARD movement of the C.P.B. from the supporting foot. A DRIVE is considered HORIZONTAL MOVEMENT (seen as level, smooth).

ENTRANCE ... Usually refers to the Choreography of the first few bars of music, prior to the actual dance routine. (Sometimes synonymous with "Intro.")

ENTRY ... A Unit or possibly a TWO UNIT PREPARATORY that precedes a specific pattern. (Usually necessary when both partners want to go into a SAME FOOT PATTERN and then follow it with an OPPOSITE FOOT PATTERN.) (See REVERSE SUGAR PUSH in CALIFORNIA SWING.)

ESSENCE ... That particular "Look" or "Feeling" that separates one dance from another. Dances can have similar CHARACTERISTICS and similar STEP PATTERNS, but without knowledge of the ESSENCE of the dance, everything could look the same. It is the ESSENCE of any dance that gives it its flavor and excitement. Isolating the ESSENCE is what many times separates the Amateur from the Professional. In learning, don't settle for less. (See "ESSENCE of CONTEMPORARY DANCE.")

EVEN UNIT ... An EVEN number of WEIGHT CHANGES. Two beats of music that start with one foot free and END with the SAME foot free. DOUBLE RHYTHM and any form of Double Rhythm (Delayed, Syncopated), are all EVEN UNITS. The other EVEN UNIT is a BLANK UNIT. ALL EVEN UNITS are interchangeable with any other EVEN UNIT.

EXIT ... May refer to the last few bars of music during which dancers end their routine by dancing off of the floor. Also, a TWO UNIT EXIT could refer to a LINK that is necessary to complete a pattern before going on to another.

EXTENDED RHYTHM UNIT ... Achieved by adding TWO STEPS to any PRIMARY UNIT.
EXTENDED DOUBLE is FOUR steps to Two beats of Music.
EXTENDED TRIPLE is FIVE steps to Two beats of Music.
There is NO EXTENDED SINGLE because it would become a TRIPLE.

FAD DANCES ... Those dances which enjoy a SHORT but widely accepted period of Dance Activity. (Usually classified in a particular ERA.) Charleston, Twist, Boogie, etc.

FLAT ... The term FLAT does not actually mean to step flat-footed. It DOES mean that we do not step TOE first. FLAT means that the entire weight is distributed over the whole foot by the time the weight change has taken place.

FLASH BREAKS — special STOPS ... POSES ... DROPS ... LIFTS (Death Drop ... Torpedo ... Freeze etc.) Dramatic pauses within the framework of the musical count.

FOOT POSITIONS ... Refers to the Basic Five Foot Positions (and their extensions).
1st ... Heels touching and toes just a thumb width apart (Feet Together).
2nd ... Feet directly apart ... A side step.
3rd ... Heel to Instep at an angle that allows both knees to face forward.
4th ... A Walking Step, one foot in front of the other, with a line thru the center of the heel and the big toe. (Walking a STRAIGHT LINE or one that CURVES either left or right is still 4th foot position.)
5th ... Toe to Heel. (Extended 5th crosses behind on an angle diagonal to 5th.)

FORCE POINT ... That part of the anatomy that initiates the action. Knowing the FORCE POINT of every move and gesture guarantees being able to repeat a well executed move.

FOXTROT ... In any given Era, the BASIC SOCIAL DANCE, done to 4/4 time, alternating or mixing SINGLE and DOUBLE RHYTHM, has been recognized as the FOXTROT of the day. There are many varieties danced at any given time, but the basic UNIT STRUCTURE is the same for AMERICAN BALLROOM, INTERNATIONAL COMPETITION, or NITECLUB.

FREE FOOT ... The foot that is moving. The one that (kicks) (taps) (touches) ... annotated by the SLASH in a UNIT.

FREE STYLE ... In DISCO, FREESTYLE refers to dancing alone. It is not uncommon for dancers to dance as a couple and then break for a few bars of FREESTYLE before resuming dance position. ... In COMPETITION DANCING, FREESTYLE is sometimes referring to the fact that there are no set SCHOOL FIGURES that must be danced. The dancers have their choice of style and routine.

GLIDE ... A smooth, projected movement, usually forward, L.O.D. with the foot barely skimming the floor.

GOLDEN STATE DANCE TEACHERS ASSOCIATION ... An Association of Teachers of Dance, started in 1963 to perpetuate and develop the UNIVERSAL UNIT SYSTEM. (Although the name is GOLDEN STATE, membership has grown to include Teachers all over the World.)

GOLDEN STATE SWING ... refers to the actual CURRICULUM of the GOLDEN STATE DANCE TEACHERS ASSOCIATION for West Coast Swing. There are many varieties and styles of West Coast Swing. The designation of Golden State clarifies those particular patterns and stylings for which GSDTA has become famous. It is totally compatible with other forms, but is more STRUCTURED in its BASICS and more CREATIVE in its development. (A very difficult dance, has now become easier to teach.)

HEEL LEAD . . . A heel lead, correctly performed, will not allow the SOLE of the shoe of the dancer to be seen. To perform this move properly, one should think of placing the FORWARD half of the heel on the floor and then transfer the weight onto the rest of the foot. Landing on the BACK of the heel inhibits body flow.

HESITATION . . . Another name for a Balance Step or a SINGLE RHYTHM MEASURE in WALTZ. Can also refer to a specific School Figure.

HOP . . . A HOP is executed on ONE FOOT. Standing on one foot, the body elevates either in place or moving and lands again on the SAME FOOT. (A HOP is shown in the UNIT SYSTEM as an OPEN CIRCLE, rather than a solid DOT.)

HORIZONTAL RHYTHM . . . Movement to a specific count either Forward, Backward or to either Side . . . The projection of the body in a smooth line. (See Vertical Rhythm.)

HUSTLE . . . A name that has been tagged on everything from a LINE DANCE to a TANGO. The late 70's will probably go down in Dance History as the HUSTLING SEVENTIES. There are also specific Contemporary dances, born of this Era. The LATIN HUSTLE, NEW YORK HUSTLE, etc.

INTRO . . . Short for Introduction. Usually refers to the TWO or FOUR BAR introduction of a specific piece of music. In choreographing, it is very popular to dance an entirely different style for the INTRO. For instance, a four bar Charleston intro before a Quickstep routine . . . or a four bar JAZZ intro for a COUPLES DISCO ROUTINE.

INVERTED UNITS . . . For the ADVANCED STUDENT of the UNIVERSAL UNIT SYSTEM. Those dances which, "BREAK ON TWO" (CHA CHA, MAMBO, SALSA SUAVE, MAMBOLERO) are best taught by INVERTING the UNIT . . . Thus the UNIT STARTS on the UPBEAT instead of the DOWNBEAT. (See Chapter on CHA CHA.)

JUMP . . . A movement whereby the body leaves the floor either STARTING or ENDING on BOTH feet.

KEY UNIT . . . The specific unit in a pattern that makes that particular pattern work. The most difficult unit in the pattern. Isolating and practicing the KEY UNIT of a pattern reduces learning and practice time.

KICK . . . Unless otherwise specified, a KICK in SOCIAL DANCE TERMINOLOGY means a movement with the FREE FOOT that is close to the ground, as opposed to a FREE SWING of the foot which swings from the hip and rises to waist height. A KICK uses the BIG TOE as its FORCE POINT, pointing DOWN for good footwork.

LATIN HUSTLE . . . The name designated for the SAME FOOT HUSTLE in California. In NEW YORK, the LATIN HUSTLE refers to the dance which is called NEW YORK HUSTLE in California. (See Chapter on various Hustle forms.)

LEAD . . . A LEAD is an INDICATION of direction . . . not to be confused with pushing or pulling.

LEAP . . . A movement whereby the body leaves the floor, starting with the weight on ONE foot and ending with the weight on the OTHER foot.

LESSON PLAN . . . The time allotment for each dance or series of classes for a given time period. All teaching should be done with the aid of Lesson Plans.

LEVERAGE . . . A term used to describe the ACTION and REACTION between two partners when BOTH are utilizing the C.P.B. rather than using STRENGTH or dancing as two separate people connected only by a hand. Correct LEVERAGE produces BODY FLIGHT.

LIFT . . . Could refer to an actual LIFTING of the partner from the floor as in an Aerial . . . Frequently used to describe the LIFTING of the C.P.B. to obtain correct posture and Body Flight. A correct LIFT leaves the shoulders free rather than rigid.

LINE DANCE . . . LINE DANCE refers to any group participation where all of the dancers are lined up doing the same routine. "SATURDAY NIGHT FEVER" was responsible for the re-birth of the LINE DANCE, which had started to die down in popularity. (1978) (See LINE DANCES under Contemporary Dance.)

LINE OF DANCE . . . Abbreviated as L.O.D. means a counter-clockwise movement around the room, as in Ballroom Dancing or Roller Skating.

LINK . . . An extra UNIT or series of UNITS that have been inserted between one pattern and another to form a particular amalgamation or to make the dance phrase.

L.O.D. . . . See LINE OF DANCE.

MEASURE OF MUSIC . . . Most SOCIAL DANCE FORMS (including Contemporary) are danced to 4/4 or 2/4 time. That is, the music is written in EVEN numbers of quarter notes. The exception is WALTZ which is written in 3/4 time. That is three quarter notes to a measure. Thus 4/4 time measures are danced in TWO BEAT UNITS (half a measure) while WALTZ is a complete measure in itself and requires two full measures to complete a basic pattern.

MOVEMENT . . . Can refer to any part of the body that moves (hand, head, etc.).

MOVEMENT UNIT . . . The actual move that takes place within the framework of a TWO BEAT UNIT. BASIC MOVEMENT refers to the action of the C.P.B. on a specific count. For instance: If the body lowers on count ONE and rises on count TWO it would be considered a DOWN-UP MOVEMENT UNIT.

NATURAL OPPOSITE . . . If reading a pattern that states only the MAN'S PART, it is assumed that the Lady's part is the NATURAL OPPOSITE. Man's part reads to step BACK, the Lady's part is assumed to step FORWARD. Unless otherwise stated, the Man's patterns will always start with the LEFT FOOT and the Lady's with the RIGHT FOOT.

NEW YORK HUSTLE . . . In this Text, the term NEW YORK HUSTLE applies to a specific RHYTHM PATTERN and all of the various RHYTHM VARIATIONS that are done in the same dance. DELAYED SINGLE ([tap] STEP) . . . TRIPLE (STEP STEP STEP) . . . and a DOUBLE (STEP STEP) comprise the pattern. It is a SIX BEAT PATTERN.

NOTE . . . Unless otherwise specified, one NOTE would refer to one BEAT or one QUARTER NOTE. (See Chapter on MUSIC.)

NOTE VALUE . . . The actual KIND of note that equals a given step. (Mainly for students of MUSIC.) One QUARTER NOTE equals ONE BEAT. DOUBLE RHYTHM is TWO Quarter Notes.

ODD UNIT . . . An UNEVEN number of weight changes within the framework of the UNIT. All forms of SINGLE and TRIPLE RHYTHM are ODD UNITS. One would use an ODD UNIT to have a different foot free. An ODD UNIT begins with ONE foot free and ends with the OTHER foot free.

OPPOSITION, Law of . . . There is a subtle force that RESISTS MOVEMENT (sometimes referred to as RESISTANCE). This LAW OF OPPOSITION states that a PULL is met with a PULL . . . and a PUSH is met with a PUSH. One presses DOWN to move UP. A SPRING ACTION is achieved when an OPPOSITION MOVE is carried to the point of being seen.

PARALLEL . . . Right or Left Parallel can be demonstrated in Dance by having partners touch the outside of one RIGHT KNEE to the outside of PARTNER'S RIGHT KNEE. The result will be RIGHT PARALLEL POSITION.

PATTERN . . . A series of UNITS that together form a specific grouping that has a NAME. In the UNIVERSAL UNIT SYSTEM we refer to a PATTERN as we would a SENTENCE. It has a beginning and an ending. The COUNT starts on the first beat of the pattern and continues to the end. It is important to know the specific number of BEATS in any given PATTERN.

PENDULUMING . . . A body so suspended from or supported at a fixed point (C.P.B.) as to swing freely to and fro using the momentum of the FORCE POINT.

PHRASE . . . Basic MINOR PHRASES are eight beats of music. Teaching or Learning to music that has SIMPLE PHRASING will help to condition the student to hear the complicated phrasing of Contemporary Music. Most SOCIAL DANCE used to phrase to counts of eight. Many Contemporary selections have an added FOUR beats or TWO beats distributed throughout the number. It is important in teaching to PHRASE OUT THE MUSIC before using a selection not familiar to you. The use of LINKS help teach the student to phrase.

POINT . . . A point with the FREE foot touching the floor with the toes. A term sometimes used interchangeably with "touch."

PRACTICAL EXAMINATION . . . That part of an exam that deals with the actual DANCING, other than the written or oral exam.

PRESS . . . Refers to the pressure exerted into the floor, pressing the balls of the feet DOWN in order to ELEVATE the body.

PRIMARY UNITS . . . Those Units which are the easiest to learn. The Units that should be learned on the first lesson. SINGLE RHYTHM . . . DOUBLE RHYTHM . . . TRIPLE RHYTHM and a BLANK. (The first five steps of every Social Dance can be learned using only PRIMARY UNITS.)

QUICK . . . A term used to denote ONE BEAT of music. In the UNIVERSAL UNIT SYSTEM we only use the term QUICK in PAIRS as DOUBLE RHYTHM. Example: a CHASSE' is a "SIDE TOGETHER" . . . TWO steps to TWO beats of Music . . . a "QUICK QUICK."

RHYTHM . . . Refers to the underlying beat of the music as it relates to the dance. Could be described as a STEADY RHYTHM, an ALTERNATING RHYTHM or could refer to a specific DANCE RHYTHM such as: CONGA RHYTHM, CHA CHA RHYTHM etc.

RHYTHM BREAKS . . . A term that has been coined to cover those variations that overlap into every dance. Various PIVOTS, GRAPEVINES etc. Most RHYTHM BREAKS are composed of DOUBLE RHYTHM UNITS and are as popular in Traditional Dance as they are in Contemporary Dance. RHYTHM BREAKS are particularly effective for forming LINKS between the various CONTEMPORARY DANCES, making the transition easier to lead and easier to follow. They are also good for CONTRAST.

RHYTHM DANCES . . . Those Dances which can be done in a specific area rather than progress LINE OF DANCE around the room. Most Contemporary Dance is classified as RHYTHM DANCING.

RHYTHM PATTERN . . . Refers to the actual UNITS that make up the Basic of a given Dance. WHIP RHYTHM in SWING is DOUBLE, TRIPLE, DOUBLE, TRIPLE (8 beats of music). NEWPORTER SALSA is DOUBLE, TRIPLE, DOUBLE, TRIPLE. The RHYTHM PATTERN is the same. The actual Dance is different because of FOOT POSITION, DIRECTION and STYLE or ESSENCE. The RHYTHM PATTERN merely refers to the number of STEPS within the framework of the Pattern.

RHYTHM UNITS . . . The BASIS for the UNIVERSAL UNIT SYSTEM. The RHYTHM UNITS are where we START. They are the actual WEIGHT CHANGES that take place for a specific Pattern. (See BASIC RHYTHM UNITS, SECONDARY and ADVANCED.)

RHYTHM VARIATION . . . Substituting a COMPATIBLE RHYTHM in a particular pattern. The LOOK and the TIMING is altered, but the PATTERN remains the same. Most of the time, what APPEARS to be a BRAND NEW STEP, is merely a RHYTHM VARIATION of something we already know. RECOGNIZING the RHYTHM UNITS enlarges our DANCING VOCABULARY.

RUMBA . . . A FOUR UNIT DANCE which alternates DOUBLE and SINGLE RHYTHM. (Can be danced starting on the SINGLE OR the DOUBLE.) Patterns for G.S.D.T.A. all start with the DOUBLE RHYTHM UNIT. At an ADVANCED STAGE, Rumba can be danced using INVERTED UNITS which will produce a "BREAK ON TWO" in the DOUBLE RHYTHM UNIT.

RISE AND FALL . . . The degree of elevation and lowering that takes place to achieve the Characteristic of a given Dance. Most easily seen in Waltz.

ROPE . . . The Street Name given to SALSA VALIENTE. The ROPE refers to the action of multiple arm wraps using Rope styling. The RHYTHM PATTERN is just a series of DOUBLE RHYTHM or MARCHING STEPS. When done properly it is a beautiful dance reminiscent of Paso Doble with a Contemporary flair. However, done WITHOUT KEEPING TIME TO MUSIC, the dance loses all of its form and style. A large percentage of the dancing public dances THE ROPE out of time.

ROUTINE . . . A series of patterns form an AMALGAMATION. Several AMALGAMATIONS, joined together with LINKS and RHYTHM BREAKS form a ROUTINE. A good routine will almost always include an OPENING, several AMALGAMATIONS, one or two HIGH LIGHTS, a CLIMAX and an EXIT. BASIC ROUTINES are a must for the beginning dancer.

RUN . . . Stepping quickly, one step after the other, with the free foot actually leaving the floor (usually DOUBLE RHYTHM in 4th foot position).

SALSA . . . Salsa means "SAUCE" and initially it referred to a type of MUSIC . . . Disco music with a LATIN BEAT. However, just as ROCK was a MUSIC before it became a DANCE . . . SALSA evolved from the MUSIC And the INTERPRETATION of that music BECAME the DANCE. There are several forms of SALSA that have evolved. SALSA PICADO (Little Triples), . . . SALSA VALIENTE (All Doubles . . . The Rope), NEWPORTER SALSA (a combination of alternating Double and Triple Rhythm), SALSA SUAVE (similar to an Open Rumba, alternating Double & Delayed Singles).

SAMBA . . . A Traditional LATIN DANCE, the Samba is a TWO UNIT PATTERN in its Basic form. The RHYTHM UNITS are SYNCOPATED TRIPLES at an advanced stage. For BASIC SAMBA it is wise to practice the MOVEMENT to SINGLE RHYTHM. The MOVEMENT UNIT is DOWN on ONE and DOWN again on TWO, with a rhythmic LILT in between. (See SAMBA and also SAMBA HUSTLE.)

SECONDARY UNITS . . . Those Units which are taught next after the PRIMARY UNITS are learned. They include: DELAYED SINGLE (a tap STEP) . . . a DELAYED DOUBLE (kick STEP STEP) . . . an EXTENDED DOUBLE (STEP STEP STEP STEP) and a BASIC HOP (STEP HOP, OR HOP STEP).

SCHOOL FIGURE . . . The School Figure refers to the PATTERN that has been selected for the curriculum that puts the BODY in the CORRECT place with the EASIEST RHYTHM UNIT and FOOT POSITIONS. Other rearrangements of the same pattern are either RHYTHM VARIATIONS or STYLE VARIATIONS.

SHUFFLE . . . In SOCIAL DANCE, a series of little steps that do not actually leave the floor. In TAP DANCING, an "OUT & BACK" move, making two distinct sounds.

SINGLE RHYTHM . . . Refers to ONE STEP to TWO BEATS OF MUSIC. Step on COUNT ONE and (hold), (brush), (kick), (touch), etc. on COUNT TWO of the UNIT.

SLASH . . . Refers to the SYMBOL on a UNIT CARD that means a KICK or a TOUCH or a BRUSH with the FREE FOOT. No weight changes take place on a SLASH.

SKIP ... Usually refers to a "HOP STEP ... HOP STEP" counted "& 1 & 2." In teaching someone to SKIP, it is advisable to start with a plain "HOP STEP." (See Chapter on teaching CHILDREN.)

SLIDE ... A Slide can be done on ONE FOOT or on TWO. It is the act of landing on the floor while the body is still moving ... and continuing to move on the floor.

SLOW ... A SLOW is ONLY USED as SINGLE RHYTHM in the UNIVERSAL UNIT SYSTEM. It refers to stepping on the FIRST beat of the Unit and staying on that foot through count TWO of the Unit.

SMOOTH DANCES ... Refers to those dances which progress around L.O.D. (Foxtrot, Waltz, Tango, Viennese).

SOLAR PLEXUS ... The location of the CENTER POINT OF BALANCE (C.P.B.) just above the navel. An area about the size of a fist.

SOLO DANCING ... Dancing alone ... as in Freestyle Cha Cha or Disco.

STAMP ... (No weight change.) Placing the foot on the floor, hard enough to make a slight sound, but still keeping that same foot free.

STANDARD DANCES ... Those dances which have withstood the test of time ... Foxtrot, Waltz, Tango, Rumba, Samba, Swing and even Cha Cha.

STYLE ... Style sometimes refers to a specific look that adds character to a Dance ... or sometimes to a Dancer.

STYLE VARIATION ... Refers to CHANGING the foot position or styling of a particular pattern WITHOUT altering the RHYTHM UNIT.

SUBTLE TRIPLE ... Those TRIPLES that are danced without being able to see or hear the obvious three changes of weight. TWO STEP is primarily SUBTLE TRIPLES (feet kept close to the floor).

SWAY ... The action of the C.P.B. with reaction from the shoulders. The C.P.B. travels to the weighted foot, and the shoulder FOLLOWS. A good SWAY can be achieved in Waltz by keepin the weight over the MEASURE FOOT. (In Foxtrot, over the UNIT FOOT.)

SWING ... The Dance that has evolved out of JITTERBUG, LINDY, NEW YORKER and JIVE. All are various forms of SWING. (Included also in this family should be the Texas PUSH and also the St. Louis SHAG.) (See Chapter on SWING ... Eastern, Western, California & Golden State.)

SWIVEL ... A SWIVEL is on the weighted foot. The heel is slightly released from the floor while the weighted foot moves from right to left or left to right.

SYNCOPATED RHYTHM UNITS ... Units that step on the "AND" count and do something else (a "tap," "kick," etc.) on the regular count.

SYNCOPATION ... The rearrangement of the regular metered beat. (See ADVANCED SYNCOPATIONS.)

TANGO ... A Standard Dance that moves counter-clockwise around the room. At a Basic Level, it is a FOUR UNIT PATTERN, consisting of: a SINGLE ... SINGLE ... DOUBLE ... and a BLANK UNIT. (Basic MOVEMENT is Horizontal, rather than Vertical.)

TANGO HUSTLE ... A Contemporary Dance which mimics the Valentino Era with Dips, Kicks and exaggerated Poses. In its Basic Form, the RHYTHM PATTERN is DOUBLE ... SINGLE ... DOUBLE ... SINGLE. It is characterized by a circular arm lead, plus a VERTICAL MOVEMENT of UP and DOWN.

TAP ... (No weight change.) A touching of the free foot to the floor without changing weight.

TEMPO ... The Speed of the Music.

TIMING . . . The ability of a Dancer to place not only the FOOT, but the C.P.B. at the precise moment as the beat of the music. Actual weight transference with syncopations, or without, that stays within the framework of the metered count.

TOE . . . A common term in Social Dance which does not ACTUALLY refer to dancing on one's TOES. TOE refers to the BALL OF THE FOOT. In describing footwork, it would be difficult to call out, "Ball of the foot, Ball of the foot." "Toe" has become acceptable for that CALL.

TRIPLE RHYTHM . . . THREE steps to TWO BEATS OF MUSIC. A LEFT TRIPLE steps Left Right Left . . . and a RIGHT TRIPLE steps Right Left Right.

TROT . . . A lilting movement of little running steps, stepping on every beat. (Heels do not touch the floor.)

TWO STEP . . . A Contemporary Dance composed of two TRIPLE RHYTHM UNITS.

UNIT . . . Two Beats of Music. (For ANNOTATION a UNIT is encased in a rectangle for easy identification.)

UNIT CARD . . . The Tools of the UNIVERSAL UNIT SYSTEM. Large Cards that represent the individual RHYTHM UNITS and/or MOVEMENT UNITS.

UNIT STRUCTURE . . . The Number and Kinds of RHYTHM UNITS in a specific Dance or Pattern in a Dance.

UNIVERSAL UNIT SYSTEM . . . The name given the UNIT SYSTEM in that it transcends Language barriers and is being taught World-Wide.

UP BEAT . . . The SECOND and FOURTH beat of Music in 4/4 time.
The SECOND BEAT of a RHYTHM UNIT.
In a WALTZ MEASURE, the Up-beats are counts 2 and 3.

VERBAL PATTERN . . . What we actually "SAY" to describe the pattern being Danced, e.g.: "Walk Walk" and "Step Three Times."

VERTICAL RHYTHM . . . The action of the C.P.B. in relationship to the legs. DOWN UP . . . UP DOWN . . . DOWN DOWN . . . UP UP etc.

WALTZ . . . A Standard Dance in 3/4 time. Waltz is counted in three beat MEASURES instead of UNITS. A WALTZ MEASURE contains ONE DOWNBEAT and TWO UPBEATS and is complete in itself.

WEIGHTED FOOT . . . The foot that receives the C.P.B. . . . the supporting foot.

WESTERN SWING . . . The name in common usage among Chain as well as Independent Studios to describe SLOTTED SWING. The Lady walks toward the Man on count ONE of each pattern, instead of rocking BACK as is danced in EASTERN SWING. (See Chapter on Swing.)

The great thing
in this world
is not so much
where we are
but in what direction
we are moving.

—Oliver Wendell Holmes

Chapter XV
MY "PEOPLES PAGE"...
(Acknowledgements)

To list all of the people who have been responsible for the growth and development of this book would be impossible. To list them in order of importance would ALSO be impossible. And so . . . listed ALPHABETICALLY are some of the people I would like to publicly thank for their efforts. They are listed alphabetically by FIRST names . . . for who ever heard of a best friend called Jones, Alice ?

A very PUBLIC but PERSONAL THANK YOU . . .

To . . . Alan and Susie Nielson for their invaluable feed-back on the use of the UNIVERSAL UNIT SYSTEM in their Dance Studio in Ventura, California.

To . . . Andrea Smith Kluge . . . our "Little Andy" in the Skippy Blair Studios for many years. Andy assisted in teachers training and was the lead dancer in most of our shows. I worked out many new dance variations by telling Andy what I was trying to achieve. I figured them out but SHE could do them!

To . . . Audree and all the gang from El Camino Press who helped get all this into print. (It wasn't easy!)

To . . . Barry Dunn . . . My professional Dance Partner when PERFORMING was as important as Teaching. Our T.V. appearances . . . SHOWS with RENE' BLOCH . . . Two and sometimes THREE shows on one week-end . . . all helped mold the ideas that have finally taken form.

To . . . Blanche Van Tilborg for seeing me thru the rough spots when I was not well . . . and for all the encouragement that kept me plugging away at the book.

To . . . Buddy Schwimmer for the 10 years (or more) that he's been part of "The Family" . . . and for the continued spread of the UNIT SYSTEM as he travels from State to State. Four time State Rock Champion & current California State Disco Champion, Buddy never stops! (Buddy owns Buddy's Dance Clinic in Costa Mesa.)

186

To . . . Bob Moen for his continued support of all my efforts. As a Swing Dancer with the L.A. Swing Club, Bob does more than his share to promote good dancing & friendship.

To . . . Carri Fox for her loyal support of every undertaking . . . for taking over my classes when the load got too heavy . . . for doing such an excellent job of helping to train new teachers . . . Carri is a real credit to the Unit System.

To . . . Carolita Oliveras for traveling all the way from Arizona on so many occasions just to help get things "rolling" with the SYSTEM . . . and THE BOOK.

To . . . Chloe Call for the many years of professional & personal association. She is an example for all to emulate when it comes to dedication to her "kids" & the Dance.

To . . . Dr. Cliff Bigelow . . . who studied with me for many years . . . for his faith in my abilities and support of my activities. (As an amateur competitor, he and his sister reached 7th in the country in International Competition). Later, as a professional, he performed in many shows & entered professional competition. Cliff & Shirley & family will always be "family."

To . . . Corky Elser for being our lead male dancer for so many years . . . and for bringing home so many awards for the system . . . Professional Latin Champion and 1st place Swing Champion with partner Sheila Blair, in 1963.

To . . . Diane and Roland Ellis, dancing friends thru the years, whose lives periodically cross with mine in the furtherance of the dance . . . and our friendship.

To . . . Dora Casares for her constant support and encouragement. She's a doll.

To . . . Gil Sais who gave us Barry Dunn and "Have Steps Will Travel." We hated to see him leave the dance profession but he is still a staunch supporter.

To . . . Jan Monan for her pioneering efforts in Bakersfield and her fantastic support and promotion of the UNIT SYSTEM. (In Niteclubs, Colleges . . . everywhere!)

To . . . Jayne Unander, noted Cotillion Dance Teacher from Los Angeles, whose well thought out questions in Teachers Training sessions were responsible for many new developments in the system. Jayne has done more to spread the word nationwide than most of us put together.

To . . . Jeanine Englehart for her constant encouragement to FINISH THE BOOK! Her untiring work with Southern California colleges have helped to spread the UNIT WORD!

To . . . Jerry Ehrhart, personal friend of some 20 years who taught the original training class that started my career in the social dance field. His poem on the UNITS is a classic.

To . . . Jim Cane who taught us all the value of a rousing support in all of our endeavors. Southern California was never the same after Jim made his home in Virginia. We all missed his "MORE MORE" at every show . . . and the excitement he carried with him for everything he touched. His DANCE MAGAZINE is read world-wide & we all feel proud to have been associated for so many years. Good Luck Jim and our best to Joy. (Mr. Cane's explanation & development of "Body Flight" is unparalleled.)

To . . . Jim Nichols for his faith in my abilities and his constant support in my activities. (like even flying us to dance camp so we would get there on time!)

To . . . John Armstrong, my oldest boy, for his thoughtfulness and his faith that "Mother can do anything!" (& love to Barbara & Johnny & Stevie from "Gramma Skippy.")

To . . . John Buckner who manages to surface every time the Association needs help. John was a top performer with the Skippy Blair Dancers for many years and we are all happy to have him back in the Association.

To . . . Johnny Luchesse for his dedication to the dance and his willingness to share his expertise whenever the need arises. Johnny is Mr. New York himself! (D.E.A.)

To . . . John Stewart, my Dad, who tap danced with me when I was only 10 . . . and who died when I was 11. He always said that if you loved the world, the world would love you back. I believe him!

To . . . Karen & Steve Allen from the Dance & Creativity Centre in Redondo Beach for all their continued support and belief in the system.

To . . . Ken Harper who has a way of making you believe in yourself. "I don't think this book would have made it without you, Ken. Here's to our continued association for many years to come."

To . . . Kenny Wetzel who keeps the TOP OF THE WEST humming and never fails to acknowledge dancers and their efforts.

To . . . Kevin Thompson, director of activities at the CRESCENDO in Anaheim for his continued support and faith in my abilities and activities, & for my designation as Chairman of judges for their $10,000.00 Competition Series.

To . . . Larry Kern who always had a way of making me feel that I could lick the world. My ideas . . . my Shows . . . my Music . . . all became strengthened with conversations with Larry. (In addition to being one of my favorite protegés.)

To . . . Lauré Haile for being an inspiration to so many teachers for so many years. Many of my own development of theories had their basis in her findings. A recipient of America's DANCING HALL OF FAME Award, Ms. Haile is known throughout the world for her teaching . . . her writing (the StepLighter) . . . her Dancing and her judging. Who could do more in the world of Dance?

To . . . Lee and Linda Wakefield who, as a dance team, have received more standing ovations than I have witnessed from any other performer. (They have appeared in many of our productions and their lift routine will be remembered as a Classic for years to come.) A special bouquet to Lee for Teaching the Unit System at B.Y.U. . . . & my fondest wish is that the whole world will one day experience the magic of Lee & Linda.

To . . . Lenore Hughes who, along with Lee Wakefield, directed Squaw Valley Dance Camp each summer. The opportunity that Summer Dance Camp presented was fantastic . . . for the dancer . . . for the teachers . . . and for the Universal Unit System. The Camp has since moved to SONORA in AUGUST and is something every dancer should experience. (Several teachers took their examination this past summer (1978) and next summer student exams will be available at camp.)

To . . . Leon Raper, founder of the Jitterbug Club of America, who went to great lengths to further the art of SWING DANCING. (Teaching for his group was a joy!)

To . . . Louis Maymon, my piano player . . . my arranger . . . my friend of some 35 years. So many years ago in Atlantic City, New Jersey . . . I sang and Louis played . . . some of the current hits of the day, but also many of my own original tunes. With Louis' patience, I learned a lot about TIMING, PHRASING and SYNCOPATION. No doubt an important cog in the wheel of the Universal Unit System . . . My eternal friend.

To . . . Lynn Vogen . . . another "family" member & one of the finest young dancers of our day. As a protegé she excelled all others in the mastery of the Unit System. Lynn did much of the pioneering work in performing arts with the UNITS and became quite adept at choreography. She won a California Swing Championship with Larry Kern . . . and the California Disco Championship with Buddy Schwimmer.

To . . . Margaret Blair. . .my Mother: On hearing someone describe the first time that they observed me with my four grown children and 3 grandchildren. . .my Mother remarked "Well . . . I started the whole thing. . . ." . . . and so she did. She not only started it . . . she pretty well kept the ball rolling. There never was an undertaking that she didn't think I could handle. (That is after we got past my borrowing the RENT money to pay rent on the local High School to produce a Show I had written in my senior year at Pleasantville High!) Her sense of humor and her utmost Faith in "The Kid" has pulled me through many a rough one. Love ya pretty lady!

To . . . Marilyn Curtiss, top dancer, teacher and super special "family" person . . . whose loyalty and dance expertise have been invaluable to the organization as a whole . . . and to me as a personal friend. Marilyn started with us as a student in 1959.

To . . . Memo Bernabei and his MEN OF MUSIC . . . who have played the GOLDEN WEST BALLROOM for the past 12 years. Memo's cooperation in the style of music for teaching . . . and the joint effort of our magnificent NEW YEAR'S EVE SHOWS (and MIDSUMMER NEW YEAR'S EVE IN AUGUST) have drawn crowds from far and wide.

To . . . Merilou Puopolo, Miss Downey 1961 and Miss Los Angeles 1963 for MISS AMERICA. It was my privilege to write the skit and coach Merilou in her talent presentation and development. WOLPER PRODUCTIONS made a TV special on the STORY OF A BEAUTY CONTESTANT which told Merilou's story . . . and filmed us in rehearsal at the studio . . . in Santa Cruz at the competition . . . & all points in between. She was the AUDIENCE FAVORITE and she was magnificent.

To . . . Mike Vander Griend, a relatively new friend who has become a permanent part of the "family" . . . a teacher at San Diego State University, Mike is currently doing a thesis on the UNIVERSAL UNIT SYSTEM.

To . . . Miles Bond, a lifelong friend who has taught all of us how to appreciate really GOOD SOUND. As sound technician for G.S.D.T.A. . . . & sound engineer for the Golden West Ballroom, he has educated all of us to HEAR and to see to it that our STUDENTS hear the best sound available. (Once you hear it right . . . you can't settle for less!)

To . . . Olen Thibideau, owner manager of the Golden West Ballroom in Norwalk, California. . . . For the continued support of the annual Dance Teachers Conferences . . . and his unending faith in my ideas, events, and accomplishments. It was Mr. "T" who first allowed us to experiment with DISCO DANCE LESSONS at the TOP OF THE WEST. They were packed & every club in the State was soon on the bandwagon. Many firsts have been accomplished at the Golden West Ballroom . . . & all thanks to "MR. T."

To . . . Patricia Armstrong Smoot . . . my number two Daughter . . . dancer par excellence . . . choreographer . . . teacher . . . and C.P.A. (can't account for that last one . . . she just happens to have many talents!) . . . Now residing in Paris, France with lawyer husband Jim Smoot, "Lucky" had frequently called from New York saying "WHEN ARE YOU GOING TO GET THAT BOOK OUT?" She and partner MIKE MIKITA won the Junior Championship at the WORLD'S FAIR IN NEW YORK IN 1964. She won many events after that, but was noted for her special performances . . . with Larry Kern, with Cliff Bigelow, with Victor Rogers, with John Buckner with Jim Cane . . . as well as dancing solo performances. Lucky would take the NEW IDEAS from the UNIT SYSTEM and put them to use even before I had a chance to test them out. Her answer: "I KNEW they would work." (Bless her for her confidence . . . and her achievements.)

To . . . Phil Martin, business manager for G.S.D.T.A. for taking so much of the load off of my shoulders . . . for helping to make the Association grow . . . and for being so absolutely dependable. Here's to many years of cooperative effort, working toward a common goal . . . BETTER COMMUNICATION IN ALL DANCE THROUGH UNIT TRAINING.

To . . . Red Rex, now deceased, who was my JITTERBUG PARTNER on the STEEL PIER in Atlantic City, New Jersey. Red was from California and together we were unbeatable.

To . . . Richard Stromberg — "just because."

To . . . Robert W. Armstrong II . . . my youngest son . . . recently graduated from McGeorge Law School in Sacramento. (I'm the only one who is still allowed to call him "Bobby.") There is no doubt that his special thoughts . . . phone calls . . . moral support in my many endeavors help to strengthen my own convictions. He knows that Mother can do ANYTHING . . . so one tries hard to live up to that!

To . . . Ruth Hood . . . (L. Ruth Hood R.N.) a very special lady who taught me that if you want something done RIGHT you have to do it yourself. She also taught me that I am responsible for me . . . that as long as we look for something . . . or someone to take care of us, we are at the mercy of the wind. Bless you for being my friend . . . my advisor . . . my own "Auntie Ruth."

To . . . Sandee Bryant Chavez . . . who gave me lessons in how to tame a tiger! Brilliant foot work as a Swing Dancer . . . great body stylist in the Latin Dances . . . and quite a personality. We all welcome Sandee to the inner circle of teaching specialists in the G.S.D.T.A.

To . . . Sandra Armstrong Brush . . . my number ONE child, with the intuition of a seer. The closeness of the past few years have made communication possible almost without words. "Sandy," Marc, and son Rick are staunch supporters of all of my efforts . . . and I of theirs. We all know that "ALL things are possible" . . . and so they become!

To . . . Shari Block who taught me how to proofread . . . and who spent several long days pouring over galleys to put the pieces together for this book. A long time friend who, with husband George, will always be a part of our "dancing family."

To . . . Sharon & Bob Boise . . . for their untiring efforts on behalf of the UNIT SYSTEM and all of the other projects that I have implemented in the past few years. Sharon has become one of the foremost teachers of the Unit System & is currently teaching for Coastline College. Bob & Sharon own "Mr. Roberts" in Newport, as well as a new large facility in El Toro. Bob travels back & forth between California and Arizona, spreading the Unit System along the way.

To . . . Sheila Blair Eglin . . . for all of her help in the past 15 years. As a new student, Sheila learned faster than anyone before her . . . and soon became a lead dancer in the Skippy Blair Dancers . . . on T.V. . . . at DISNEYLAND . . . and in clubs all over Southern California. California LATIN AND SWING CHAMPION in 1966 with partner Corky Elser . . . headliner in LAS VEGAS with partner Larry Kern . . . Sheila made the dance world sit up and take notice! Recently, she has assisted in taking over classes so that I could be free to finish . . . the BOOK! . . . another loyal forever family member.

To . . . Tom Boots, personal friend, President of the L.A. SWING CLUB and a prime mover in the final "getting the book done" phase. My thanks to both Tom and Bev for their efforts in behalf of all dance. They give much time to make life more enjoyable for those who dance.

To . . . Tom Mattox . . . owner of the SUNDANCE STUDIO in Downey, who has probably done more than any other person to demonstrate the effectiveness of the UNIT SYSTEM. From Club dancer to owner of one of the most qualified and successful Dance Studios in Southern California in less than a year, Tom attributes his knowledge of dance to the UNIT SYSTEM. He teaches in SEVEN NIGHT CLUBS in FIVE NIGHTS as well as running the studio. (which boasts a staff of all G.S.D.T.A. qualified teachers.)

No doubt I have momentarily forgotten someone who should have been included in my list of important people in my life. It seems that everyone I meet contributes substantially to my own development or that of those around me. If I have forgotten you . . . I love you ANYHOW! . . . and God Bless.

"THE WRAP UP"

I really can't believe this is finally happening. We're actually going to press. I must share my feelings with you of this past few weeks as we neared press time. It made me think of the first time I made RICE. It seemed so simple, but I finally wound up with three pans . . . and there was still more rice to go. WELL . . . that's where I've been. No matter how many pages I finished, it always seemed that there were "just a few more" to go.

In the final days, there have been moments of "you gotta be kidding!" where you finally decide that the whole thing was too much in the first place and "STOP THE WORLD . . . I WANTA GET OFF." But there are people around like John and Richard . . . and Max, who printed our pictures in the middle of the night. There are also thoughts of people who somehow missed the "peoples page" but whose contribution was really worthwhile . . . people like Tony Peeden who spent a whole year helping the Association grow . . . and Marci Miller who first inspired me to open my own studio . . . And Mr "J" who managed the Studio for quite a few years and contributed much time & effort to all of us. I'm sure there are more because everyone I meet contributes something to my life. I wish I could thank them all.

The final "letting go" of this book is like giving birth to a baby . . . one that I've been carrying for twenty years. I believe I've left a little bit of me on every page . . . so treat this book gently. The UNIT SYSTEM is something that will grow from year to year, just as a child grows. Share that growth with me. Let me know your experiences with the system. Perhaps you too can contribute to its growth.

Sincerely, yours for better dancing

Skippy Blair

The G.S.D.T.A. sends qualified UNIT SPECIALISTS all over the country . . . to colleges . . . teachers seminars . . . dance workshops etc. There are programs for every age group and every level of performance. If you would like to receive information on any of the following subjects STATE the information you desire and tell us your area of interest.

- Unit Cards
- Teachers Training
- Qualified teacher location
- G.S.D.T.A. membership
- Future Publications
- Teachers Newsletter
- Lecture series
- Shows and/or Special Choreography

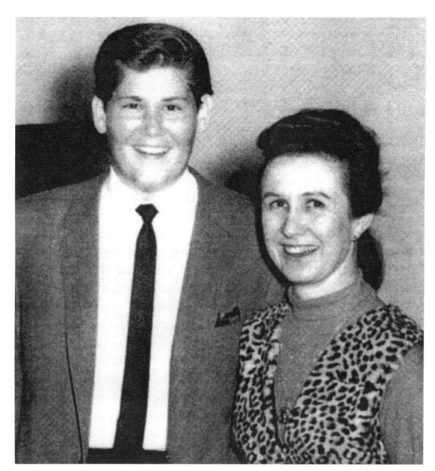

Wayne Newton & Skippy Blair, at Skippy's Studio in Downey, CA 1965.

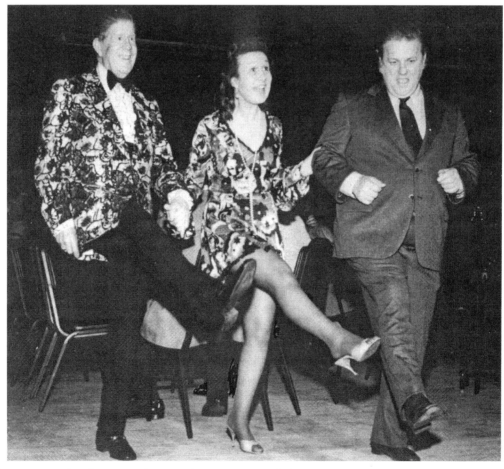

Rudy Vallee, Skippy & Charles Durning at the opening of the Stardust Ballroom in Hollywood in the 1970

PHOTOGRAPHY CREDITS

H. LEE HOOPER for pictures from 1959 to 1965 (Miss Downey photographer)

LUCILLE STEWART 1966 to 1968 (Nationally known dance photographer)

TRINI CONTRERAS 1969 to 1971 (official Miss California Pageant photographer)

JOHN MARTIN 1973 and 1974 (Los Angeles Dance photographer)

PHOTOS BY "KELLEY" 1976 and 1977 (Golden West Show shots)

GREG PFRUNDER 1978 official photographer for G.S.D.T.A.

MR. CARTER (Social Dance shots at the Golden West Ballroom in Norwalk)

RICK MALMIN (Cover photo of Tom Mattox and Susanna)
DONNA ORTLIEB (Studio Photos of Lynn & Buddy)

SPECIAL THANKS to

The DANCE SPECIALISTS . . . Teachers . . . Teacher Trainees . . . and Students who posed for over 500 pictures during the picture taking sessions. All of the dancers are G.S.D.T.A. associated . . . from:

SUNDANCE STUDIO in DOWNEY

MR. ROBERTS STUDIO in NEWPORT BEACH

DANCE & CREATIVITY CENTER, REDONDO BEACH

. . . and MORE THANK YOU'S

To all of the organizations, groups, clubs, schools etc. that have made the UNIVERSAL UNIT SYSTEM spread so far . . . so fast:

- B.Y.U.
- U.C.S.D.
- Cal State Fullerton
- Coastline College
- Golden West College
- Orange Coast College
- Modesto Junior College

- Long Beach State
- O.L.P.H.
- San Diego Swing Club
- Bay Area Dance Clinic
- Golden West Ballroom
- New York State University
- P J's in New York

(and . . . "We've only just begun". . .)

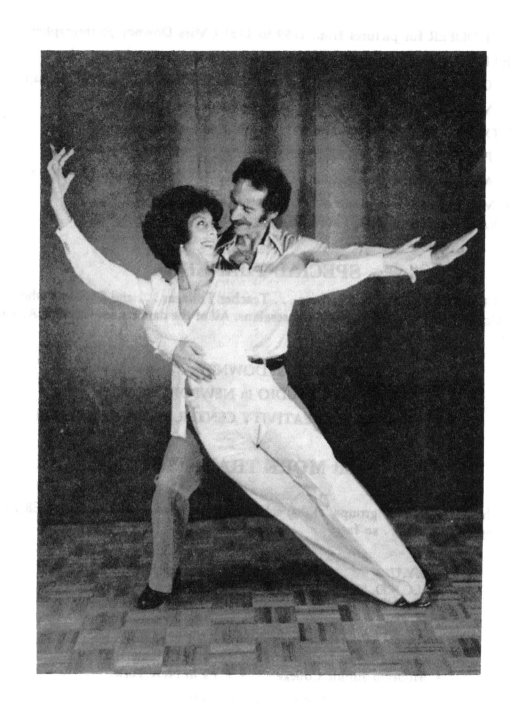

BOB AND SHARON BOIES
NEWPORT BEACH, CALIF.

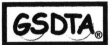
Straight Count: e & a 1 e & a 2   *(Marching, Straight Count)*
Rolling Count: & a 1   & a 2   *(Rhythmic, Rolling Count)*

The most difficult concept about counting seems to be the confusion over where the *&-Count* and the *a-Count* take place. Look at the *Count* shown above. Note that the *&-Count* and the *a-Count* are NOT located in the same place in *Straight Count*, as they are in *Rolling Count*. Frequently, people will call the *Straight Count* - leaving out the "e" and assume they are using *Rolling Count*. **Location - location - location!** The difference is tremendous. The practice of calling out "1 a2 - 3 a4" really produces *Straight Count* dancing from both the caller and the dancer. The mind does not distinguish between "1&2" and "1a2."   The rhythmic call of "&a1&a2 - &a3&a4" allows the **Center Point of Balance** to OWN the "&"-Count.

Practicing *Rolling Count* develops a habit that allows you to control the body, not only **prior** to the weight change, but actually before the *Receiving Foot* leaves the floor. That action produces an upper level, rhythmic body flow. Leaving out the *&-Count* makes it more difficult to move the *CPB* before stepping. *Straight Count* usually produces movement that comes from the legs or the hips, rather than from the *Center*. The opposite extreme: *Counting* "e&a1e&a2 - e&a3e&a4" is a **busier form of Straight Count**, but is still *Straight Count*. It has a tendency to make the dancer look busy, rushed and **slightly ahead of the music.**

This article was written in answer to E-mails and personal discussions with dancers who are serious about working toward an upper level degree of timing, and from judges who are frustrated with watching a high level of "hitting the breaks" coupled with a low level of timing. My answers are based on a compilation of notes from Intensives and Judging Seminars over the past 3 years. **Results of Critiques show that the body flow of a dancer can be greatly improved simply by changing the way the dancer *Counts*.** The evidence is overwhelming. Swing dancing is continually reaching higher levels of performance. It is important to explore every possible technique that will teach newer dancers how to keep better time to music.

Musicians actually play *Straight Count* when it is called for. (After all, not all music is written to be dance music.) However, musicians that make us feel like dancing are the ones who play with *feeling*. They are the ones who **make** you want to dance. They bring life to the Music. They bring life to the Dancer! Musicians who are not **born** with that ability, actually **learn to feel the music,** simply by applying *Rolling Count.* to what they already play. The **feeling** behind great swing music is the musician's ability to read *Straight 4/4* time music, and actually **swing** that music by applying "*Rolling Count.*" **The result is music that inspires us to dance.**

Some dancers are born with that talent - an inborn feeling for timing, rhythmic expression. and what we refer to as *"Measured Movement."* They are one in a thousand - but the other 999 of us can **learn** to feel those same things by dancing to a *Rolling Count* (which puts the magic in the music.) AND, even more important, the dancer can learn to supply that feeling, even when the music being played is not all that great. **Many dancers today can actually make you hear things in the music that you did not know were there.**

Here is an experiment for developing a "feel" for Rolling Count: Here is a simple syncopation that most dancers use in West Coast Swing. The "Call" is: " & Step Kick & step Cross." The moves takes place on "&a1 &a2." Try dancing that syncopation using a Straight Count: "& 1 & 2" or "e&a1 e&a2." Both are Straight Count. So far, we haven't found anyone who can make that one work. Give it a try and let us know your results. **Rolling Count is the real answer to an advanced level of performance..**

GSDTA®

Skippy Blair © 3-92 Rev. 10-96, 3-04, 4-04, 1-05

Salsa, like Swing, was once simply a word, used to describe a specific kind of MUSIC. Much Later, it became a dance. In the late 1970's, several different kinds of Salsa emerged. Salsa MUSIC covered a wide variety of tempos and sounds. The textbook "*Disco to Tango and Back*" has one of the most comprehensive breakdowns of that era for Salsa. Extensive, on site research, (several months) identified several different forms of Salsa, which were then categorized according to tempo and style.

Salsa Suave - The smooth 8-*Beat* rhythm that has changed only slightly since the '70's, is still easily recognized as "The" Salsa of today. This is the form that many people still confuse with Mambo - simply because of the similarity of **floor pattern**. However, when you start to isolate the differences, you find that there are several. Salsa is a Level One Dance - danced with an upright posture, prancing attitude and an elegant stride.

Salsa Picado - This series of little tiny Triples is frequently misdiagnosed as Cumbia. This has been a popular dance form in metropolitan areas, starting in the late 1970's.

Salsa Valiente -Two Hand Salsa, popular in the 70's, stepped on every beat of the music. Today, we call that dance "Melange" because it changes the look when you change the music. This dance has been a popular form of social dance in every country and every community for as far back as we can trace. This *Two Hand Rhythm Dance* feels like marching and takes on the look of Swing - Hustle - Salsa - or whatever music plays. Today's *Salsa Valiente, in some circles* is being classified as *Merengue*. The only similarity is the *Rhythm Pattern* of the dance.

Salsa Suave (or just plain **Salsa**)

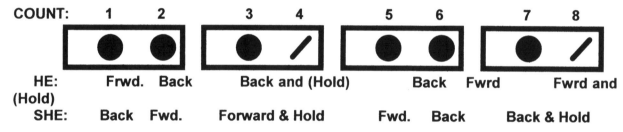

COUNT:	1	2	3	4	5	6	7	8
HE: (Hold)	Frwd.	Back	Back and (Hold)		Back	Fwrd	Fwrd and	
SHE:	Back	Fwd.	Forward & Hold		Fwd.	Back	Back & Hold	

In SALSA, the forward & back *Breaks* occur on *Counts* "1" and "5". There is an air about Salsa that carries a proud attitude of assurance and elegance. The *Posturing* is delightful and the *timing is held in control by holding the "4" and the "8".* I*In* MAMBO, the Forward & Back Breaks are on *Count* "2" and *Count* "6" = a pushing action which sends the body in a new direction.

Mambo can be danced to *Salsa* Music, but It does not FEEL the same. *Cha-Cha* can be danced to *Rumba* music. *Mambolero* can be danced to *Rumba* music. However, dancing the same dance to different music, does not change the name of the dance.

Here's a little test.: Turn off all the Music. You should be able to identify the dance being danced, when no music is playing. When a dance is performed at its peak level of performance, an observer can almost hear the music - even when there is no sound. When no music is playing and someone dances Salsa, it does not look like *Mambo*. It is not simply the same dance breaking on a different beat. Each dance has its own unique style and essence.

"*Mambo Kings*" may or may not be remembered as an important movie, but the Dance is an important part of social dance history. *Mambo* has been around since the 1940's and hit peak popularity in the early 1950's. Today, *Mambo* dancers range from New York to California (with a heavy concentration in Florida.) This fast paced Latin Dance is the forerunner of Cha-Cha.

Today, in 2005, the NEWER Mambo Dancers are asking questions like "Does Mambo have to *Break* on "2" ? The answer is a resounding "YES!". MAMBO has fast changes of direction (Breaks) on *Counts* "2" and "6". Authentic Mambo requires lots of body control, shine moves, and ripple action.

Salsa **has similar patterns - a similar look - but an entirely different FEELING.** An untrained eye easily mistakes one for the other. Teachers learn to recognize the similarities of any dance and then they isolate the differences. **It is those differences - NOT the similarities - that allow us to discover and appreciate the Essence of every dance.**

Mambo **has an "8-*Beat*" Basic Pattern.** HE always *Breaks* Forward with his Left foot on *Count* "2" and *Breaks* Back on his Right Foot on *Count* "6". SHE dances a *Natural Opposite*.. She always breaks Back on her right foot on count "2". She breaks Forward on her left foot on count "6" **The Basic Rhythm Pattern for Mambo is:**

	Delayed Single	**Double**	**Delayed Single**	**Double**
Count:	1 2	3 4	5 6	7 8
He:	Lift Break F.	Back Back	Lift Break Bk	Frwd.Frwd
Foot:	(L) L	R L	(R) R	L R
She:	(Lift) Break B	Frwrd. Frwrd	(Lift) Brk Frwd	Back Back
Foot:	(R) Right	Left Right	(R) Right	Right Left

2005 Update Note on SALSA: Today the teaching of *Salsa* has progressed to a point where we seldom hear the old count of: "123 and 456." Counting weight Changes can work at a basic level, but counting actual beats of music allows for a higher degree of musical interpretation. The closer we get to counting **real musical count**, the more the dancers will be on time with the music.

There are 8 *Beats* of music in a Salsa pattern. It is important to know what is taking place on **every one of those beats** of music. Learning to PULSE any dance adds an extra dimension. SALSA pulses the "3" and the "7". By lifting and accenting count "3" and relaxing on "4" - a pulse is created that acts as a heartbeat to the dance. This pulse repeats itself ,accenting count "7" and relaxing down on count "8".

At a more advanced stage, many dancers do a tiny kick on "4" and "8". In order to really FEEL the pulse of Salsa, try tightening up all of your muscles on count "3" and again on count "7". (Say to yourself the "3-4" and the "7-8". You will be amazed at the feeling of power that comes through the body.)

Skippy Blair, National Dance Director 𝕲𝖔𝖑𝖉𝖊𝖓 𝕾𝖙𝖆𝖙𝖊 𝕯𝖆𝖓𝖈𝖊 𝕿𝖊𝖆𝖈𝖍𝖊𝖗𝖘 𝕬𝖘𝖘𝖔𝖈𝖎𝖆𝖙𝖎𝖔𝖓, is current Education coordinator for the World Swing Dance Council. Ms. Blair is the originator of the **Universal Unit System®**, a popular training method for dance teachers, taught in Universities and studios world wide. www.Swingworld.com is our Website. **Dance Dynamics® and GSDTA are located** at 12405 Woodruff , Downey, Ca. - For information, please call: 562-869-8949.- or Email: Skippy@Skippyblair.com

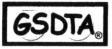

Skippy Blair © 10/98, Rev. 1/03, 8-03, 12-04

Once throught of as a difficult dance to learn, West Coast Swing has become easy to understand through the use of the *Universal Unit System*® Anyone who can dance *Triple Rhythm* (3 Steps to two beats of Music), can learn *West Coast Swing* in just a few lessons. Even if you have had trouble with *Triples*, learning the *Universal Unit System*® can make easy work of dancing a "Triple" and easy work of learning this exciting "California Dance."

People respond well to simple rules when learning any new skill. Explaining all of the possibilities in ANY dance, makes the dance sound complicated. When teaching **basic math skills,** we don't talk about fractions and decimal points. We concentrate on learning to count - to add and subtract. That lays the foundation for future learning.

Include in Lesson One:

Our first introduction to *West Coast Swing* is teaching a *Triple Rhythm Break*. By teaching *Triples* only, the student learns to stay *Centered* over the right foot for a *Right Triple* and centered over the left foot for a *Left Triple*. This allows the dancer to start feeling where each individual *Rhythm* starts and ends. The student soon learns to **distinguish a *Left Triple* from a *Right Triple*.** This all takes place on lesson #1.

Followers are taught that they will start every pattern with their *Right* foot by walking forward on *Count-1* and *Count-2* of EVERY pattern. Followers soon learn what to do on *Count-1* and *Count-2* of **every pattern** that they are going to learn in their first series. This simple statement gives the dancer confidence, just owning that piece of knowledge.

Leaders are taught that they will start every pattern with their Left foot on *Count-1* -*by stepping* in the direction that he wants the follower to go. If she is facing him, his first step will be back. If she is behind him, his first step will be directly forward. Many times, on *Count-2*, his RIGHT foot simply returns to where it was before *Count-1*.

The next most important piece of knowledge, is how to ***Anchor***. **Each partner learns that Counts "5&a6" of a 6-Beat pattern, is an *Anchor Triple*.** HE keeps his right foot behind his left foot and SHE keeps her left foot behind her right foot.

Let's review the simplicity of this process. The Follower knows to walk forward on *Counts* "1-2" of every pattern and to end each pattern with a *Left Triple*, (At basic level, a *Triple Rhythm Anchor* takes place on every "5&a6" of a *6-Beat* pattern.) That only leaves the foot placement of the followers *Right Triple*, on *Counts* "3&a4" to deal with. Simply stepping three times (Right & Left Right) for *Counts* "3&a4" - while keeping an eye on your partner, really works.

A verbal *Call* of "WALK WALK &a STEP 3 times and an ANCHOR in place" usually has a new dancer feeling comfortable and confident on the 1st lesson. The Follower is also taught to keep their CENTER (Center Point of Balance) and their eyes, facing their partner.

The Leader learns to stay centered to his partner as he does his *Back Rock* or *Forward Rock* (according to the location of his partner.) He has learned to *Anchor in place* on *Counts* "5&a6" of every "6-Beat" pattern. The "Call" for his *Left Triple* is simply: "STEP and TOGETHER FORWARD" - (a *Left Triple* on *Counts* "3&a4".)

In lesson #1 - GSDTA suggests teaching a **Triple Rhythm Break**, a **Left Side Pass**, and an **Underarm Turn**. They are taught in that specific order to facilitate learning. However, once learned, the sequence is changed in order for the student to become familiar with the sound and the feeling of ***musical phrasing***. Level I Music is appropriate for teaching Level I Patterns.

Phone: (562) 869-8949 Email: Skippy@Swingworld.com Website: www.Swingworld.com

Level I Music starts with two *Sets-of-8* as an introduction, followed by a series of four *Sets-of-8* that is usually repeated four times before starting another major phrase. The dancers are given the following sequence which is a total of **32 Beats of Music**:

- **2 Left Side Passes** (12 Beats of Music)
- **2 Underarm Turns** (another 12 Beats of Music)
- **2 sets of Triple Rhythm Breaks** (8 Beats of Music)

This beginning amalgamation, repeated over and over, soon becomes routine. This first lesson establishes both **Rules of Movement** and **Rules of Timing**. By repeating the Four "*Sets-of-8*" the dancer starts to recognize when a phrase in the music is going to end. The student soon learns that a new sequence starts over on a new phrase. Understanding this concept establishes a confident feeling of accomplishment and makes the dance seem fun and easy.-

It is exciting to see a student's eyes light up when they first feel the music and the dance come together. In addition to being a great learning experience, this **Lesson One** has also been FUN - mainly because it worked. The educational experience is evident when the student has learned to understand the following terms: **Centering - Sending Foot - /Receiving Foot - Left Triple** and **Right Triple**. The student has also begun to feel the connection between the music and the dance. By using phrasing in the teaching, the student learns to feel the points where new phrases begin and end.

Progressing through the First Basic Series

Each subsequent lesson should add only one new pattern - but rearranges the sequence, in order to keep the lesson moving, and exciting. By staying with the **basic Rhythm Pattern of Double, Triple, Triple** for the 1st Series of lessons, the student becomes familiar with *body placement* and *leverage* and becomes more sensitive to how the dance relates to the music.

Learning **Rhythm** and **Style Variations** at a future time is much easier when the student has learned all of the Basic "*6-Beat*" *Patterns* using that consistent **Rhythm Pattern** of **Double, Triple, Triple**. This method of teaching is part of the **Universal Unit System®.** It's main focus is based on creating a strong connection between body movement and the music. Staying with one *Rhythm Pattern* allows the new dancer to absorb other elements while drilling the foundation upon which future lessons can be built.

2007 NOTE: Jordan Fresbee and Tatiana Mollman are teaching all over the world, and have had a FIRST PLACE winning streak for several years. They have won every major West Coast Swing competition that exists, and have become the torch bearers for GSDTA and Dance Dynamics. The recent TV Show, "So You Think You can Dance," also contributed to West Coast Swing fame when **Benji Schwimmer,** took First place and his **counsin Heidi** was in the top ten. Benji's father, **Buddy Schwimmer** was part of our original teachers training in the 1960s and early 70s.

If you are studying Disco to Tango & Back you are learning the UNIVERSAL UNIT SYSTEM and Dance Dynamics, and you are well on your way to becoming a very knowledgeable dancer. Good Luck with your dance expeience.
